Eyes Wide Open

"By situating the body (or *soma*) right at the center of sitting meditation practice, Will Johnson helps initiate a quiet, slow revolution. . . . Such a contribution to meditation instruction is transformative in numerous respects. This book, like previous books by the author, is a landmark text in the contemporary literature of homecoming."

JAMES MARTIN, COFOUNDER OF
MINDFUL SOMATICS INSTITUTE

"With his delightful stories and exploration of the many wisdom traditions, Will Johnson continues to impress upon us the importance of the embodied experience. If we are to gain any traction on the spiritual path or to address that 'nagging inkling' that something just isn't right in our lives, this little gem of a book can guide us. Johnson offers many simple techniques to do this, honing in on vision as the vehicle for our exploration. The daily experience of 'looking' has been imbued with the power of transformation with one quick read! Will Johnson continues to be at the forefron* *f body-based dharmic practice and its confluence witl

JACKIE A
ADJUNCT FACUL'

Eyes Wide Open

Buddhist Instructions on Merging Body and Vision

Will Johnson

Inner Traditions
Rochester, Vermont • Toronto, Canada

Inner Traditions
One Park Street
Rochester, Vermont 05767
www.InnerTraditions.com

Library of Congress Cataloging-in-Publication Data

Names: Johnson, Will, 1946- author.
Title: Eyes wide open : Buddhist instructions on merging body and vision / Will Johnson.
Description: Rochester, Vermont : Inner Traditions, 2016. | Includes index.
Identifiers: LCCN 2016005305 (print) | LCCN 2016006953 (e-book) | ISBN 9781594770005 (pbk.) | ISBN 9781620551561 (e-book)
Subjects: LCSH: Spiritual life—Buddhism. | Meditation—Buddhism. | Vision—Religious aspects—Buddhism.
Classification: LCC BQ5660 .J64 2016 (print) | LCC BQ5660 (e-book) | DDC
    294.3/444—dc23
LC record available at http://lccn.loc.gov/2016005305

Printed and bound in the United States by Versa press, Inc.

10 9 8 7 6 5 4 3 2 1

Text design and layout by Priscilla Baker
This book was typeset in Garamond Premier Pro with Avante Garde and Kinesis used as display typefaces

To send correspondence to the author of this book, mail a first-class letter to the author c/o Inner Traditions • Bear & Company, One Park Street, Rochester, VT 05767, and we will forward the communication, or contact the author directly at **www.embodiment.net**.

To the seer and visionary in all of us

Contents

when my mind was cleansed of impurities
like a mirror of its dust and dirt
I recognized the Self in me

deep in my looking
the last words vanished

joyous and silent
the waking that met me there

LALLA

if you use your mind to look for Buddha
you won't see Buddha

to find Buddha
you have to see your nature

BODHIDHARMA

with my eyes wide open
I absorbed everything
as a sponge absorbs liquid

HENRI MATISSE

The Monk Who Lost the Contest

right behind your eyes
you *are there*

Take a moment, and you can feel yourself there. Looking. You're always there, and whenever your eyes are open, you're always looking. So intimate is your connection with your looking that when you say, "I'm looking," you're not just saying that you're engaged in the act of seeing. You're also implying that you *are* your looking, that how you look and what you, in turn, see are a direct reflection of who you are in this moment.

No matter what its contents may consist of, the visual field only ever offers us two choices, two different ways of looking and seeing, and the choice we make profoundly affects how we experience ourselves in this moment. It all happens in the space behind your eyes, the place from which you look, the place where awareness of self and awareness of vision cross paths.

Ordinarily the way we view the visual field confirms in us a felt sense of separation from everything we can perceive to exist outside our bodies. The visual field that I look out on, with its infinitude of multiple, discreet objects, with its convincing sense of *otherness,* is so *out there,* outside of myself, and I am so *in here,* right behind my eyes and inside my body. This way of seeing and being—through which I experience myself as somehow poured into my body, like a beverage into a bottle, and view everything inside my body as exclusively *me* while everything outside my body is *other than me*—effectively splits the whole of experience into two neatly separated worlds—one inside, the other outside. And even though these worlds are constantly interacting with each other, still they must remain forever separate and disjoined. This is, far and away, how most of us view the world and our relationship to it.

But this splitting in two of the world of experience—into an inside-the-body world of thoughts, sensations, feelings, and personal identity and an outside-the-body world dominated by the otherness of the visual field—creates in many of us a lurking uneasiness and tension, a sense of isolation and loneliness that we're not easily able to shake, a feeling of alienation and disconnection from the larger world into which we've been born and out on which we look. This subtly pervasive sense of separation, of vague disconnection—mind separate from body, self from other, inner from outer—is at the base of the human condition, and it's staring us in the eye. We may have no idea what it is we feel that we're splitting ourselves off from. All we may sense is that something just feels . . . a bit off. Something keeps tugging at us, some niggling little feeling (or perhaps not so niggling and not so small), and even though we've accepted it as part of being human, it still doesn't particularly feel very good.

The Buddha spoke of this uneasiness, this nagging inkling that something isn't quite right, as *duhkka.* The great thirteenth-century Sufi mystic and poet Rumi spoke of this uneasiness as well, in terms completely resonant with how split in two your world of experience can be carved by this way of seeing. He would say it makes you feel separated from something you very badly want to reembrace and that feeling separated in this way hurts, both in your body and in your soul.

As common as it may be, this isn't the only way we can look out at the world. There's a second choice we can make, and it's almost the exact opposite of the first. Instead of reinforcing how isolated and alone we are in this vast universe, the visual field is equally capable of reflecting back to us a felt sense of connection and inclusion, as though it were offering an invitation to merge with the energies of the larger universe in which we live and look out on, rather than confirming how irrevocably separated from them we are.

Through the shift in perspective of this second kind of seeing, divisions between your inner and outer worlds start to drop away and you begin, bodily, to experience an intimate connectivity to the world you look out on. Instead of a world composed of an infinite number of separate objects, of which you are but one, you become privy to a substratum of experience—what mystics have often referred to as the great ground of being—that underlies the world of appearances and ties all the individual parts back together into a single, cohesive piece. Beyond the mind caught up in conventional divisions of inner and outer, there's another place of perception that you can directly access, a place of far greater ease and profound relaxation in which you no longer feel so disjoined from the world you see.

However, even though it's freely available to everyone, the reclamation of this unified perspective still has to be earned.

If you feel drawn to its perception, you will want to shift your relationship with the world you look out on, transform the way you look and see—consciously, intentionally, and altogether naturally—so that what you see supports your participation in this more connected state, rather than your continued estrangement from it. And that's what this little book hopes to show you how to do.

Fair enough, but the challenge that literally faces us as we work to shift our relationship with vision is that, even though we have our eyes open, we don't necessarily see what's here to be seen. As Anaïs Nin famously observed, "We don't see things as they are; we see things as we are." We don't just look out on the visual field with the impartiality of a mirror. Instead, we interpret. We filter out. We sift through and sort. We project. We view the visual field through a distorting lens created by our personal biases, beliefs, tensions, hopes, fears, and prejudices. If the lens is powerful enough, it can color everything that we see.

The anatomical structures associated with vision—the eyes with their retinal openings, the cones and rods that register color and light, the neural pathways and electrical impulses that transmit visual data to the visual cortex of the brain where it's all somehow reassembled into a recognizable image—are like the neutral components of a shutter on a camera. But then each of us goes and places our own unique lens over that shutter, and our choice of lens manipulates and colors what we ultimately see.

How are these filters and lenses formed? Often our conceptions and beliefs about how reality is constructed are so powerful that we're unable to have a direct perception of what we're actually looking out on without immediately and automatically applying this conceptual overlay and buffer. As just one example, we believe that physical objects are solid and inert, so we tend to see them that way—lifeless, motionless, and inanimate—but by the end of this book the solid, blank wall that you look over at on the far side of the room might start looking quite a bit more alive and shimmery (but let's wait and see).

It's not just the attitudes and beliefs in the mind that create these filters and distorting lenses. We also create them through the way we live in the body. A body that is tense will view a world on constant alert. A body that is sluggish will view a world of depression. A body that is angry will keep encountering situations to be angry about. A body that is relaxed and balanced will view a world of grace and beauty. A body under the enchantment of love can sometimes possess the uncanny ability not to see any of the flaws and shadows of its object of affection.

But if we're not seeing things as they truly are, and if seeing and being are so inextricably reflective of each other, then we can't be experiencing ourselves as we truly are either and must be putting up instead with a version that is distorted and less authentic than it could be. If we're looking out on the world through a distorting lens of beliefs, prejudices, and patterns of bodily tension, we're also distorting who we, the lookers, believe and experience ourselves to be. The task and path of the Buddhas has always been oriented toward helping us come out of the dreams of who we think we are and awaken into our true, essential nature. If we're to apprehend this essential nature (and wake up from the nightmare of separation in the process), then it would make sense that we would want to cleanse our vision and remove whatever distorting lenses we've superimposed onto our perception of the visual field.

The Theravadin Buddhists have a beautiful word for this clear vision that allows us to experience ourselves as we truly are. They call this way of seeing and being *vipassana,* which translates as "seeing things as they are." And to learn to see things as they actually are, not just as we perceive them to be through our multiple filters of distorting attitudes and bodily tensions, is the intent and purpose of their practice.

The perfect symbol for this extraordinarily clear visioning is a clean and polished mirror that reflects whatever is set in front of it. A mirror has no biases or prejudices. It doesn't interpret what it sees; nor does it project its own beliefs out onto the world it reflects. It makes no distinctions or valuations. It has no preferences. It simply reflects back what's here to be seen. Here's what the Sufi poet Rumi had to say about the visioning of the mirror in contrast to the way in which humans mostly look and see:

> the mirror can reflect every face as it is
> because it has no face of its own
> the mirror neither fawns over beauty
> nor turns away from the homely
> beauty appears on the face of the mirror
> so does homeliness
> the mirror has no quarrel either way
> but a pleasant image comes to your eyes
> and you become happy
> a homely image comes
> and you become withdrawn

The clearer we're able to keep our vision and the fewer the layers of reactive grime on the windows through which we look out on the world, the closer we get to the truth of who we are. So . . . how can we keep the windows reasonably clean? How can we look out on the world through eyes that mirror, rather than interpret or project? How can we shift our vision so that what we look out on heals, rather than reinforces, the separation?

To better understand how to create this mirrorlike vision and way of seeing, let's turn our attention for a moment to a multigenerational tale of succession that began in the time of the Buddha and ended in an extraordinary contest that took place in the mountains of China over thirteen hundred years ago.

Toward the end of his life, some twenty-five hundred years ago, the Buddha decided he wanted to choose a formal successor, someone who so understood and embodied the teaching that, after the Buddha passed away, he or she could be relied on to keep the teachings alive, their pure essence intact, and to resolve any questions or disputes that might arise. As we will see, there are many different ways to choose a successor.

In the case of the Buddha, he sat silently and twirled a lotus flower before a throng of seated students who had come to hear him speak. Every morning, without fail, he would come out from his living quarters, sit down, and explain the teachings to whoever had come to hear. But on this morning, he did something completely out of character. After sitting down, he didn't say a word. He just sat there, twirled the flower, and looked out over the assembly, moving his gaze from one person to the next.

Most of the students may have felt a bit nervous and confused by his strange behavior, but one of the senior students,

Mahakashyap, realized the exquisite humor of the situation and burst out laughing. After all, the truth that can be spoken of is only words; the silent truth that can be recognized in the moment of the twirling of a flower is what we're really after. Mahakashyap couldn't contain the joy of his insight (and may have found the nervous response of the rest of the assembly quite funny as well). It is said that the Buddha *looked* at Mahakashyap, which is when his student broke into laughter. The Buddha simply smiled back and declared him his successor.

Over the centuries, in an unbroken chain, the process would be repeated. The person who had been charged with preserving the essence of the *dharma*, the teachings, would choose a successor before he passed on.

Around the year 500, the twenty-eighth successor of the Buddha, the Indian prince Bodhidharma, traveled to China, where he continued the ritual of naming a successor to whom the teachings could be entrusted before he passed away. This move from India to China ushered in a whole new era in the transmission of the Buddhist dharma. Bodhidharma was given the title the first patriarch, and from one person to the next, successors kept getting chosen until we finally find ourselves, sometime around the middle of the seventh century, at the monastery on Huang Mei Mountain, where the fifth patriarch Hongren was living and teaching. And here our story can begin in earnest.

One day, toward the end of his life, Hongren announced that a contest would be held to determine his successor (no twirling flower for him!). The rules of the contest were simple: write a *gatha*, a poem, that demonstrates your understanding of the essence of mind. And the prize was tantalizing—the composer of the best poem would become the sixth patriarch and would be entrusted with the promotion, preservation, and protection of the dharma.

At first, it didn't appear as though it would develop into much of a contest. At the time of Hongren's announcement, there was a head monk living in the monastery whom everyone greatly admired and looked up to. The name of this monk was Shenxiu, and while Hongren held the title of the fifth patriarch, Shenxiu was entrusted with much of the teaching and explication of the dharma that took place at the monastery. So prominent and admired was Shenxiu within the organization of the monastery that all the monks simply assumed that he was the only one qualified to write the poem and be named the sixth patriarch. And so no one bothered to write a poem of his own but simply waited to see what Shenxiu would compose.

They did not have long to wait. In the morning, Shenxiu's poem had been posted on one of the monastery walls. It read simply:

> *the body is the tree of awakening*
> *the mind is like a clear mirror*
> *at all times we must work to keep it polished*
> *and not let any dust collect*

The appearance of the poem in the early morning hours created a great stir within the monastery. When Hongren was told of it, he immediately approved of the wisdom it contained.

"Practice according to this poem," he is said to have told the assembly of monks. "Not only will you receive great benefits, you'll avoid falling into any traps or mistakes. So go, light incense, and pay respect to this poem. Keep reciting it, explore what it's telling you, and you're bound to see your essential nature." Clearly, Shenxiu was to be given the robe and begging bowl that would signify that he was the successor to Hongren.

Ah, but not so fast. Now there was another lowly, mostly unnoticed monk living at the monastery named Hui Neng. As a young man, he happened to overhear a Buddhist discourse and simply by hearing the words experienced a profound understanding and awakening. He heard of Hongren and was determined to study with him.

When he finally arrived at Hongren's monastery, he was able to arrange a meeting with the patriarch, who immediately challenged him in his understanding of the teachings. Hui Neng had been born into a lower-caste family from the south, and Buddhist teachings at that time were generally reserved for the upper, more educated classes. As a test, Hongren taunted Hui Neng, asking him how an illiterate barbarian from the southern countries could possibly understand the dharma teachings of the Buddha. Hui Neng calmly replied that, although there was a great deal of outward difference between himself and Hongren, their essential nature was one and the same. Hongren recognized that Hui Neng possessed an unusual, innate understanding of the dharma and accepted him into the monastery but assigned him a low-ranking job in the kitchen so as not to attract attention or arouse any jealousy amongst the older, more class-conscious monks.

Hui Neng saw the poem that Shenxiu had composed and decided that it didn't satisfactorily explain the essence of mind; in fact, it didn't speak of it at all. Rather, it spoke only of the practices that lead to a realization of one's essential nature, so he decided to compose a clarification of Shenxiu's effort.

Unable to write himself, he requested the help of a friend in the monastery, and by the next morning the following poem had appeared on another monastery wall:

there's really nothing like a tree of awakening
nor is the mind anything at all like a mirror
since everything is eternally empty of any
*   fundamental essence*
where could dust collect

Well, you can imagine what kind of stir that created.

Later that evening, Hongren summoned Hui Neng to his chambers, where they spoke at length of the nature of mind. While Shenxiu's poem beautifully and simply presented the path of practices that leads to an awakening of essential nature, Hui Neng's response captured the essence of what that indescribable nature is like. Hui Neng was named the sixth patriarch and the shocked community of monks loyal to Shenxiu had to deal with the reality that their favorite son had lost the contest.

Ours is a world that is unkind to losers. The word itself carries a heavy, pejorative weight. Touch the wall at an Olympic swimming final one-hundredth of a second after your competitor and you're relegated to the status of an also-ran, a loser, and your efforts are looked down upon as somehow inferior and failed. While outwardly Hongren had praised the wisdom contained in Shenxiu's poem, inwardly he may not have been completely satisfied. Yes, the poem perfectly described the practices, but Hui Neng was right: the contest had called for a poem that portrays the essence of mind, not the practices that lead to it. One may know the practices and follow them, but that in itself is no guarantee that the person has completely realized his or her essential nature, and only to someone fully realized could the dharma robe and bowl that signify the succession of the teaching be awarded. Hongren had little choice but to award the prize to the one who embodied the dharma, rather than to the one who was the master teacher of it. And so, while students of Buddhism continue to be intimately familiar with the story of Hui Neng and routinely praise the wisdom in the poem he composed, Shenxiu and his poem tend to be more overlooked, even forgotten, relegated to the historical bin of those who came in second. Shenxiu is mostly remembered, after all, as the Monk Who Lost the Contest.

But clearly, Shenxiu was no dunce. In four short lines, he managed to enunciate a path of practices that leads to a profound shift in how we view reality, and the subsequent development of Buddhism in China and, later, in Japan reflects the ongoing dialogue and tension between his and Hui Neng's poems and their two different approaches to the teachings.

In Hui Neng we have the example of the person who's fully realized the indestructible nature of mind that doesn't require any practices or techniques as support. In Shenxiu we have the example of the dedicated practitioner who's always on the alert, always watching the moment-to-moment changing show of mind and body, always aware of when one's lost one's awareness, always gently bringing the mind and body back to a condition of watchful awakening, always keeping the clear mirror of the mind as free of dust and obscuration as possible. Hui Neng describes what the enlightened state is like, but Shenxiu shows us the way to create the conditions in which Hui Neng's understanding might dawn on us. If you had to make a choice, which is ultimately the more valuable and useful to you at this moment: a description of your destination or a map of how to get there?

For the purposes of understanding our relationship to the visual field and the world in which we live, I choose Shenxiu. His poem is a shorthand manual on how to initiate mirrorlike vision and provides a number of direct clues to help explain how we can contact our essential nature through embracing the visual field and merging with it, rather than viewing it as something alien and separate.

The foremost clue that Shenxiu gives us is that the body plays a critical role in supporting the ability of the mind to function like a mirror and see things as they are. For most people, spiritual practice is primarily an examination of what we conventionally call mind; body is often overlooked as a lesser partner in the exercise. But Shenxiu is telling us that this isn't so. In fact, quite the opposite is true—for our minds to become awakened and start functioning like a mirror, rather than a constant interpreter or projector, we first need to awaken the body. What might this mean, and how do we go about doing that?

Then, by referring to the image of the mirror as the symbol through which to understand the workings of the mind, Shenxiu acknowledges the primacy of *vision* in the pantheon of our senses. After all, a mirror is about vision, pure and simple. A mirror reflects what is visually apparent. To create a mind like a mirror without obscuring layers of dust and soot is, literally, to *see* things as they are. What happens when we let go of the thoughts and interpretations and analyses and projections? What happens when we awaken our body, silence our thoughts . . . and see?

ONE

Awakening the Body

the body is the tree of awakening

Shenxiu's poem begins by telling us that the body is the tree of awakening. It does not say the tree of the wish-fulfilling jewel, the tree of the fruit of life, the tree of restful dreams, the tree of abundance. It says the tree of awakening. What happens at that tree is an awakening, and the awakening needs to occur in the body.

But what's so sleepy about the body? And what needs to wake up?

The body has fallen asleep through our having lost touch with its feeling presence, its palpable, organic, felt life, its vibrancy so deeply sourced in sensation. We lose ourselves in thought and tense ourselves in ways that hold this vibrancy in and stifle its emergent, felt glow. It's as though we've turned down the dimmer switch on the body's felt presence, just as a nursery school teacher will dim the lights when it's time for the small ones to take their nap, and in the darkening that's ensued our bodies have become very sleepy indeed.

And so the first thing that Shenxiu tells us is that, in order to contact our essential nature, we need to wake the body up.

14

We need to rekindle its felt presence, nudge it gently out of its sleepiness (again like the kindly nursery school teacher), and welcome it back into a more wakeful state.

To awaken the body is to awaken the long-dormant tactile sensations that fill the body from head to foot. So small, oscillating so fast, these minute little pinprick blips and wavelets of sensation, once awakened, can be felt as part of a massed flow or current, a felt shimmer, vibrating lightly here, surging strongly there, pulsing, throbbing, dancing, effervescing throughout the entire body.

Simply by placing your relaxed awareness in any part of the body, sensations that have long been asleep, in a kind of hibernation, mostly unfelt and blanketed over, can start to wake up. They begin to hum, throb, pulsate, to come back to life, and this vibratory tingling, this sparkling into wakefulness, can be immediately and directly felt.

Sensations are the flowers on the tree of awakening, in constant bloom as the body wakes up to itself, one bursting cluster after another, lightly buzzing here, suddenly cascading there, tingling, vibrating, a current of flow, nothing unmoving or solid, like individual droplets of water in the current of the life force that flows through you like a stream through a meadow.

But while sensations can be felt to exist everywhere in the body, we ordinarily have little awareness of them. Ours is a strongly disembodied, even somatophobic, culture and we suppress the feeling presence of the body. We hold sensations in and, in doing so, dull them. We blanket them over and hold back their glow. We value *psyche* over *soma*—the life of the intellect with its abilities to formulate abstract thought and linguistic concept over the body with its singular ability to feel. And yet it is the simple sensory field of bodily sensation that Shenxiu points to as the source of an awakened knowing that can lead us out of the muddle that layers of abstract thought have so successfully built up around us.

For the body to awaken from its dreamy sleep, sensations need to be allowed to come out of exile, pardoned for crimes they never committed, welcomed back into the cloth of awareness, given permission to once again make their shimmer felt. Suppressing the natural condition of the body's felt shimmer, we're mostly only aware of isolated pockets of pain, generalized unpleasant sensation or large-scale numbness, and the occasional rush of bodily pleasure, fleeting as it may be. And so, Shenxiu tells us that we need to awaken the slumbering body and reembrace the whole extraordinary field of sensation, every bit as major a sensory field as the fields of vision and sound, but one to which we mostly remain blind and deaf, literally out of touch.

To better understand the mechanisms that keep sensations so sleepy, it's helpful to examine the relationship between body and thought. The sensational presence of the body remains dormant, unfelt, and asleep as long as we stay lost and adrift in unbidden thought, consumed by the story lines that the mind incessantly spins and pours out, like some feverishly active, linguistic version of a silkworm. If we're really honest in examining what's actually happening to us at any given moment, we quickly realize that a large portion of our moment-to-moment experience is taken up by the domineering presence of the internal, mostly involuntary, monologue of the mind, the silent voice inside one's head that keeps speaking and making pronouncements about incidents, events, people in our lives, feelings, fantasies, perceptions, fears, regrets, hopes.

Sometimes this monologue sounds like a play-by-play sports announcer, describing in detail our every move, our every scored goal, our every dropped ball. Sometimes it's more like a political commentator, analyzing and explaining what's going on in our life, exploring the situations and causes that have led to this moment, offering predictions of what's likely to follow as a result (and not infrequently spinning the news, like the silkworm again, to support a particular ideology). Sometimes the monologue criticizes, judges, admires, or makes comparisons with the behavior of others. Sometimes it gets completely caught up in the drama of our personal lives and story lines, our excitement and despair.

Our unbidden thoughts gravitate strongly to playing back events that occurred in the past and to looking forward to events that are yet to come. What they're incapable of accessing, however, is an awareness of what's actually happening to us right now, in this very moment. And this is where body comes in, for this is what body is so adept at doing. Sensations are so evanescent, so transitory in appearance— arising and passing away, appearing and disappearing with such rapidity—that we can only be aware of them, only feel and know them, right now and it is this ever-morphing realm of right now that the Buddhist dharma is so interested in exploring. Past and future are places in the mind; right now is the felt experience of the body.

The relationship between sensations in the body and random thoughts in the mind is an uneasy one at best. Mostly, the relationship is like a teeter-totter: when one side is elevated, the other is suppressed. It's not possible to be lost in thought and present in body at the same time. At those moments when we drift off into internal monologues, we block out and lose awareness of body as feeling presence. It's as though the appearance of unbidden thought—the ongoing chatter of the internal, involuntary monologue—has a numbing effect on sensation. Lost in thought, you lose awareness of body.

The teeter-totter needn't be stuck in this one place, though. It can shift position, and suddenly what was elevated drops down and what was suppressed rises up. While it is true that lost in thought, we can't be present in body, what is also true is that once we allow sensations to be fully stirred and kindled (what the great twentieth-century Burmese vipassana teacher U Ba Khin referred to as "activating *anicca*," kindling an awareness of body as a field of constantly changing, shimmering sensations), once we let ourselves feel body, once we bring it back to life, awaken it from its slumber . . . in that moment unbidden thought stops.

In an awakened body, consciousness will naturally function more like a mirror. Random thoughts and entrenched beliefs create the dust that Shenxiu refers to later in the poem, a kind of obscuring coating, a filmy layer that keeps the mirror of the mind cloudy and the sensations of the body blanketed over.

So either you're lost in your mind or present in your body. You can't be both at once. When there's a great deal of semiconscious monologizing going on, mind serves as a barrier that separates the visual field that you look out on from the place in the center of your being out from which you're looking, and so you reinforce your sense of being separate from the universe in which you live. When you're able to kindle awareness of body as a unified field of shimmering, vibratory, tactile sensations and energies, the barrier starts dissolving and the place from which you look and the visual field out on which you look start merging back together into a more unified, coterminous phenomenon.

How do you feel sensations? How do you let their presence emerge? How do you welcome them back into felt awareness? How do you help them wake up?

The most powerful thing you can do is simply give yourself permission to feel them and then turn your attention to them. You can't force them into appearance. You can't manufacture or create them. Even though you may not be aware of them, they're still here *in potentia* all the time, like an object waiting patiently in a drawer you rarely open, and you can't create something that's already here.

Even though our culture may have a strange bias against doing so (and as ludicrous as it feels to even have to say this), know that it's completely okay to open to the feeling presence of the body. It's okay to let sensations come forward into feeling. It's okay to surrender to their organic current and presence, giving yourself permission to feel their vibrancy and life, shedding the taboo that, for whatever reason, our culture has placed on their awareness. And it's also okay, even sublimely natural, to enter into the condition of consciousness that felt presence reveals.

First you invite them back. And then you turn your attention to them. By focusing your attention on any small part of the body, sensations that have taken you up on your welcoming gesture naturally start surfacing, like stars coming out in the early evening sky. Keep allowing sensations and turning your attention to them, and more and more keep emerging until, one day, the sky of the body, like a view of the Milky Way on a clear night in a remote desert, is filled full with them. Remember: we're only unaware of them because our attention is elsewhere. By simply turning your attention to them, you shine a warming light on them and they begin to wake up and come out of their shadowy slumber. They sparkle, they tingle, they shimmer.

One of the many remarkable tenets of twentieth-century physics suggests that there's no such thing as completely objective observation. As soon as you turn your attention to something, you somehow start affecting what you've turned your attention to; something in your focus starts interacting with what you're focusing on. In the case of sensations, as soon as you start paying them attention, they respond by waking up and coming back to felt life.

While it may take time and consistent effort to become fully conversant with the felt range of sensations throughout your body, just letting yourself feel the body right now—this giving permission to sensations—is as sophisticated a strategy to awaken them as anything. Some of the sensations in the body may feel achy, others numb. Some may feel tingly and fizzy, like a carbonated beverage. Others softly shimmer, as though the body were emitting a natural glow. Some feel very good. Others hurt. All of them are your body.

The good news is that sensations can be aroused, resurrected, woken up from their long sleep, welcomed back into the fold of direct and immediate experience after their long ostracism. The even better news is that we needn't do anything heroic to nudge them back into felt awareness. We just need to turn our attention to them.

Meditations to Awaken Feeling Presence

Bringing Sensations to Life

So . . . just let yourself feel.

Begin by turning your attention to a small area at the top of your head about the size of a large coin. Just let yourself feel whatever it is you can feel here, in this one little part of your body. A subtle tingling? A buzzing perhaps? A pain or pressure? Something stirring, moving even? Just let sensations be, as they are. No need to change or alter them in any way. No need to make them stronger or weaker than they are. To awaken the body, individual sensations need to be accepted exactly as they're first felt.

As soon as sensations appear, like stars coming out at night, they start flickering and percolating, changing their form, massing together like starlings in flight, streaming along as part of a larger current. Because they're so individually minuscule and flicker on and off with such rapidity, they appear more as a phenomenon of flow than as discrete entities. In this sense, it's more helpful to think of *sensation* not as noun, but as verb. Not as individual object, but as process in eternal flux.

Be patient. Sensations are there. Let them come to you. You can't rush them. You can't force them to awaken. They wake up at their own pace, but the relaxed focusing of attention on them starts rousing them, warming them, inviting and calling them back to felt life.

Slowly start spreading your awareness across and over the entire area of your scalp. Spread your awareness slowly, just the tiniest little bit of movement from one place to the next. What do you feel as you move your attention in this way? A shimmering, a light tingling, a buzzing, an aching, a throbbing, a pulsing, a pressure, a kind of tickling? The sensations may be so light as to be barely perceptible, or they may be as strong as a rushing current in a stream—so much going on in so small a space, every single little blip of sensation apparently arising out of nowhere, disappearing just as rapidly, constantly reappearing, constantly passing away again, constantly changing.

Next spread your awareness over your face, very slowly again, part by little part. Feel what's going on in your forehead—minute individual blips of sensation massing together into a common current. Sometimes you may be able to name a sensation: achy, tingly, heavy, itchy. At other times you may be aware of a feeling quality for which you don't have any words to describe. It doesn't matter. Just feel what's here to be felt, exactly as it is. No need to name it, and certainly no need to change it, to try to make it feel a certain way. By letting sensations come to awareness and then accepting them exactly as they are, they start to shift and change spontaneously, on their own. What's been hidden gets revealed, and whatever needs to be resolved gets swept up in the flow.

Keep spreading your awareness around your face. Feel into your eyebrows. And then feel into your eyeballs. When you become lost in thought, your eyes lose awareness of feeling presence. By waking up the sensations in your eyes, letting them come forward and be felt, unbidden thought melts away, right before your eyes.

Feel your nose, every little part of it, its long shaft and both individual nostrils. Spread your awareness to include the sensations in your cheeks, your temples, your jaw. Just feel them. And if, by feeling sensations, they start to change, just let them.

Move your attention to your mouth, your lips, your teeth, your tongue. Feel your chin. Feel your ears. Feel the entire head as a unit. From the outside looking in, it might look like a solid object, but from the inside feeling out, it's just sensations and wavelets, streaming and flowing, a tactile river in flux.

In this way, keep moving your awareness, part by part, through your entire body. Feel your neck and throat, your shoulders down into your arms, your elbows, your hands, each individual finger. Become aware of the feeling presence in your upper torso, starting perhaps at the top of your chest and moving down the front of your entire ribcage, rib by individual rib, deep inside into the diaphragm itself, following around the sides of your upper torso, continuing around the back of your rib cage until you come to the spinal column, and then move your awareness from one vertebra to the next, feeling everything. If you come across an unexpected sensation of strong discomfort, take an equally strong inhalation right into the sensation. Relax as much as you can as you exhale.

Feel your lower torso in the same way, the front of your abdomen, the sides of your belly walls, your lower back, and lower vertebrae.

Open to an awareness of the sensations that form your entire pelvic basin. Moving your attention slowly, feel how the texture and tone of sensations can subtly change from one small place to the next. Let yourself feel into your organs of elimination and reproduction.

Move your awareness down both of your legs, your upper legs, your knees, your lower legs, your feet, every little toe. In the beginning, move your awareness down each leg separately. As you become more adept at feeling sensations, you can start passing your awareness through both legs simultaneously.

When you feel particularly distracted in your meditation or your movements through life, it's helpful to pass your awareness, slowly, part by part, through the entire body. As mind settles and body comes more vibrantly to life, it then becomes easier to feel the entire body all at once, as a unified field of feeling presence. Once that global awareness fades or becomes again more diffuse, you can then go back to taking a tour of your body, part by individual part.

Moving your awareness through your entire body, letting yourself feel the sensations that are your body, is the basic technique of the medical body scans that are so successfully being promoted in hospital mindfulness programs. It's also the central practice of the powerful Burmese forms of body-oriented vipassana meditation. The more you pay attention, the more sensations appear. The more you can feel the entire body as a field of shimmering, tactile sensations and wavelets, the more awakened body becomes.

Constantly moving your awareness through your body—like an art connoisseur perusing every square inch of a masterpiece—keeps body from falling back into a dreamy, unfelt sleep. So whether you're sitting on your cushion in meditation, driving your car, or pushing a buggy through a supermarket aisle, keep remembering to feel. Never avoid a part of your body. Never jump over an area of unfelt presence. Do your best to feel everything, every little cell, strong or weak, and appreciate how everything keeps changing. The awakened body is like a river, its sensations constantly streaming, constantly moving. The slumbering body is more of a stagnating pond, its sensations numb, heavy, hardly showing up at all.

Opening the Portals of the Body

Alternately, you might want to take a more circuitous route through the body during which you focus your attention successively on specific points, or portals, in the body. Start by letting yourself feel two areas on either side of the spine at the level of your lower back. It doesn't matter how big or small they are. Just settle your awareness in these two locations and relax into, and let yourself feel, whatever's there to be felt.

The more relaxed attention you pay to these places and the longer you're able to stay softly focusing on them, the more sensations are likely to emerge. Take your time. You may want to spend several breaths exploring each of these portals. You may want to spend several minutes.

Once you've been able to kindle awareness of feeling presence in these two spots, start moving your attention slowly upward, on either side of the spine. Feel how sensations get stimulated in the parts of your body you're passing over as though little feet were walking along these parallel pathways. Keep moving your attention upward, until you bring it to rest in the back of the shoulder, in the middle of either shoulder blade. Just open to the sensations, feeling whatever it is you can feel in these two locations of the body.

Next, pass your awareness down through the sensations on the inside of your arms, all the way down to your hands, and let your attention come to rest on the inside of both wrists. Passing your awareness from portal to portal stimulates sensation as you go. Once you've arrived at the portal, just settle in, rest, and wait for sensations to come streaming forward.

Once you've clearly registered and explored sensation in your wrists, move your awareness back up the outside of the arms, all the way over the shoulders, and let it come to rest at the next portal on either side of the spine, at the juncture of the upper back and lower neck.

Let the two spots merge into one now as you move your attention up the back of the head, over the crown of the cranium, and let it come to rest at the top of your forehead, where your skin meets your hairline. Let yourself feel the sensations right at the surface of your forehead as well as deep inside the middle of the cranium.

The single spot breaks into two again and starts moving downward, hugging the contours of your face, your chin, your throat, spreading itself downward until it comes to rest as two spots on either side of your sternum at the level of the heart. Let yourself open to the full range of sensations, space, and energies that you can feel at this place in your body.

And then keep dropping down, down the rest of the rib cage, down the abdomen, until the two spots come to rest on either side of the front of the pelvis. Take some time as you explore these spots, and then drop down even more as your awareness passes down the front of your legs to come to rest on the outside of either ankle bone, just a bit behind and beneath the protruding bone itself.

To complete the circuit, pass your awareness up the back of your legs slowly so you can register the quality of sensations over which your attention is passing, over the buttocks, and let your attention come to rest on two spots on either side of the spine at the level of the lower back, the place where you began. And in this way, you complete one circuit through the body.

Each of these places in the body may reveal very different qualities of sensation. Some may feel completely impersonal with little or no emotional tone attached; others may feel intensely moving and poignant. Some may feel strong and surging in their presence; others may feel much subtler, almost imperceptible. As you pass your awareness through your body in this way, it's not as though you ever lose touch with the sense of the whole body. It's just that the individual places you're focusing your attention on form the temporary center of the whole body.

Constantly moving your attention—either in a relatively straight line from the top of the head to the bottom of the feet, or through following a more roundabout circuit like the one just described—keeps body alert and awake. When you can feel body all at once as a unified field of shimmering tactile sensations, do so. Whenever your awareness starts wavering, whenever unbidden thought sneaks back in, whenever you become distracted or agitated, remember to move your awareness again through your body in an intentional manner, part by part, feeling whatever's there. Watch how the activity of the mind calms down, at times even stopping or dissolving, as you keep passing your awareness throughout your entire body, waking it up as you go.

Every one of these points is like a portal, or gate, into the mystery space of your body. At first, what emerges through these portals is pure sensation: vibrating, shimmering, tingling. As you keep a relaxed attention on each individual portal, the sensation may start becoming gradually more translucent, and then each portal may start ushering you into a feeling awareness of the vastly spacious nature of the interior of body. Each portal can then become a gateway into the ground mystery itself—the substratum of being in the very center of our center where our individual separateness dissolves and we enter back, no matter how momentarily, into an embodied awareness of the nondual state, the place that Rumi referred to as union.

After you've become aware of each of the portals in sequence, you may choose to make another circuit through each of them in turn, or you may choose to feel all of them simultaneously. Feeling all of them at once strongly awakens the body, not just at the portal itself, but in the spans between the portals as well.

Sometimes you can easily locate the portals, but other times you may have to let go of your expectations, relax your awareness, and explore the area to find out where the particular portal actually exists in your body. For example, sometimes the back of the shoulders will include an opening through the front of the shoulders as well. Sometimes the two areas at the juncture of the upper thoracic and lower cervical spines merge and expand to include the whole of the back of the neck or even the whole of the back of the head. Sometimes the portal in the forehead can be felt more palpably in and through the eyes themselves, out through the top of the head, or down into the throat. Sometimes the portal at the front of the chest can be more easily found as a single point rather than as two separate spots. Just relax, let go, and find what you feel.

The order of the portals is quite simple: lower back, back of the shoulders, inside of the wrists, back of the neck, forehead, level of the heart, front of the pelvis, outside of the ankle bones . . . and back up to the lower back.

While contacting the quality of mind that is very much like a mirror is the topic proper of the next chapter, awakening the body to full awareness of its felt sensational presence is the prerequisite that allows that quality of mind to emerge. Rumi is quoted as saying, "Dissolve the body into vision; become seeing, seeing, seeing!"

If we want to create a mind like a mirror, we need to dissolve the body into vision, to merge its feeling presence with the visual field that you look out on. And if we wish to dissolve the body into vision, we first need to awaken it from its slumber of numbness, from its suppression of sensation, for how could we possibly dissolve the body into vision if we're not even able to feel it?

TWO

Mirror Bright

the mind is like a clear mirror

Ordinarily we take the visual appearance of the world we look out on so completely for granted that we lose sight of any participatory role we might play in its creation. We believe that visual appearance is an intrinsic property of physical objects, that the visual field looks the way it looks whether we're looking at it or not, that it exists completely independent of any act of vision on our part. But. . . .

If a random event occurs and no one's there to *see* it (the age-old tree crashing down in the philosophical forest), has anything that we conventionally refer to as *visual* occurred?

You may have been a sophomore in high school when a teacher first asked you about the *sound* falling trees made in a distant forest with no one around to hear it. Grudgingly and probably after much harrumphing (I mean what a ridiculous question, really!), you were forced to admit that, okay, while *something* can be said to have occurred, it couldn't properly be labeled as *sound*. For sound to occur, three conditions have to be present: a source of friction that generates soundwaves; the presence of a functioning ear in the near vicinity (and not just a human ear; animals, birds, and insects are all equally capable of hearing sound); and finally, the wide-awake consciousness, directed toward listening, of the sentient being to whom that ear belongs. If any one of these three conditions is absent, sound doesn't occur.

That much most of us can understand. It becomes far more uncomfortable, however, if we apply this same line of reasoning not to sound, but to vision. If no one was nearby in that forest when the tree fell over, did its dropping to the ground exist as a *visual* event? And just as you concluded that no sound could have occurred if no one was there to hear it, and for the exact same reasons, it couldn't have occurred as a visual event either *if no one was there to see it.*

For better or worse, we'd like to believe that the world we live in is like an eternal, preexistent stage set on which we play out our lives. But while most of us would agree that the objects of the world clearly exist on some sort of physical level, whether or not anyone's looking at them, they must exist in a form somewhat equivalent to soundwaves that, on their own, don't constitute sound. Light waves bombard and crash through the universe constantly and incessantly, but only as energetic waves, invisible until or unless someone looks at them and then—and only then—do they burst forth into visual appearance, and then only for as long as that someone keeps looking at them. When it comes to our participatory cocreation of the visual field, the New Age trope *we create our own reality* couldn't be more accurate. The world you look out on only looks the way it looks because you're looking at it, cocreating its visual appearance as you do.

What a magic show, this dazzling display of appearances! "Now you see me," says the visual field, "now you don't. But you can never know that you don't, for as soon as you turn your eyes to what, a moment ago, had no visual appearance, now it does!"

The first two components of the act of seeing are almost always universally present. First, there are the visible waves of light that physical objects emit. Second, there are your eyes and the complex physiological miracles and mechanisms that allow you to receive and recognize these waves. The wild card is the third component, the consciousness that is both awake and focused on the action of seeing. And here's where *how* you look not only colors what you see but affects who you are in this moment of looking.

Most of the time, we have our eyes open but don't really see what's here to be seen. We find ourselves pulled away from vision into thought. We become distracted and don't really look where we're going (most of the time we get away with it, sometimes we stumble). And rarely will we go anywhere near accepting responsibility for being cocreator of the visual field. After all—or so we want to believe—the visual field is eternally out there, just as it appears whether I'm looking at it or not, so why all this fuss about exerting myself to *see* it with precision and clarity, like a mirror, in its richness, its rainbow of colors, its subtle nuances, no distortions, exactly as it is?

Through equating the essence of mind with a clear mirror, Shenxiu provides the answer: reinvigorate your looking so that what you see is actually what's here to be seen, without distorting filters or concealing curtains, just as a mirror reflects whatever's placed in front of it, and then you can more easily settle into the quality of mind about which his teacher had challenged the monks of the monastery to write the poem of succession.

Lost in thought, we don't just lose touch with body. We don't see clearly either. Unbidden thought, self-image, and the physical tension that accompanies them not only stifle and blanket over the feeling presence of the body. They also create a metaphorical layer of dust over our lens of vision that both obscures the mirrorlike essence of mind at the core of our being and distorts the appearance of the visual field out on which we look.

Most of the time, the conventional mind functions as interpreter or projector. Relying constantly on language to formulate its intentions, mind tends to demand that we identify ourselves with the speaker of all its thoughts, whom we all refer to as *I*. That, says conventional mind, is who you are. Mostly what *I* does is to look protectively after what it believes to be itself. It wholly and completely identifies that self with the object of its physical body (even though it goes nowhere near actually experiencing what that body feels like) and looks out on the world outside the body in terms of potential benefits and threats.

Its first function is as interpreter. How do *I* make sense of what's happening in my immediate vicinity? Is there threat from a bear nearby? Is there presence of an attractive mate? How can *I* then manipulate this situation to *my* advantage? How can *I* both benefit and protect *myself* (meaning, again, the physical body that is dimly perceived as object but not directly experienced as field of sensations)? Our interpretations are highly subjective and depend entirely on the lens of beliefs that we superimpose on the act of seeing.

Then, after a while, mind might start turning into a projector, quite like the projector in the cinema that is able to create a fantasy scene right before your eyes. Projection too is largely a function of the lens that has been placed over your eyes through which you view the world, and this lens is both created and reinforced through the unique holding patterns of tension in your body. Angry people look out on a world of anger. Sad people see misery everywhere. Arrogant people see opportunity and potential to manipulate. Predators see prey. An old Indian saying tells us that when a robber meets a saint, all he sees are his pockets.

The mind as projector sees what it most wants to see, and the price it pays for this manipulation is that it often gets disappointed, or in trouble, when reality-as-it-is turns out to be different from what mind had so unwittingly projected. Mind, of course, does many things, but mostly these are its two primary modes—as interpreter and projector—and you can hear the internal commentary in one or the other of these modes going on constantly in your head in the form of the silent monologue that no one but you can hear.

But a mirror? A mirror is the exact antithesis of both interpreter and projector. A mirror reflects whatever's in front of it. With no prejudices. No judgments. No interpretations. And absolutely no projections. In other words, with no thought forms or story lines with which to interpret or project and create a layer of distorting dust over the clear essence of the mind.

Fair enough. But why is Shenxiu so insistent that if we want to contact the quality of mind that behaves like a mirror, we first need to awaken the body?

Without the liberation of feeling presence throughout the entire body, mind naturally gets caught up in the parade of its ongoing internal monologue with its interpretations, projections, and self-images. If you suppress the felt presence of body, you feed the mind that interprets and projects, and then not only do you create a split between body and mind, you also create separation between yourself and the world you look out on.

Rumi tells us that there are two ways of looking and seeing—through the eyes of the head or the eyes of the soul. The eyes of the head look out and see a world from which they feel separated. The eyes of the soul look out upon that same world and feel a palpable, underlying connection to it. The eyes of the head support thoughts in the head. The eyes of the soul witness a place beyond thought. For Rumi, soul and the felt experience of body are deeply interrelated—different ways of pointing to the same phenomenon. The more you awaken the felt presence of the entire body, the more you become immersed in soul.

Shenxiu is telling us the same thing; if we want to contact mind's essential nature, we will want to start *seeing* not just with our eyes but with our whole body, and we'll want to look out on the world through a lens of vision free of filmy residues of thought dust, just like a clean, bright mirror.

So . . . as you look out on the visual field, let go so completely of whatever tensions you feel in your body and mind that the visual field starts flooding into you, like a tsunami of love, and *you* are swept away and disappear. Your conventional sense of self—the image in your mind you hold of yourself, of who and what you believe yourself to be, and the thoughts that support this identity of separation—can get washed away and a different quality of self, so empty of substance, yet full of presence, aware of the currents of the life force that flow everywhere and connect everything, can start coming forward as your more natural state.

Shenxiu reveals a great secret in his poem: the way to contact your essential nature is to see with your whole body, opening fully to vision while simultaneously feeling your entire body, head to foot, every little cell of it, leaving nothing, no little part, out. From the perspective of essential nature, the feeling presence of body is as integral a component in the act of vision as are your eyes.

For a mind to function as a mirror, two things are necessary. First, every little part of the body needs to be inclusively felt. A mirror doesn't just reflect objects on some parts of its surface and not others. The visual field bonds with the mirror everywhere on its surface with no little part left out, and the same is so for the body. Feel every little part of the body so the visual field can properly reflect on every little part of the mind. Remember that body—not just your eyes—is your organ of vision.

Second, the mirror needs to open its reflecting embrace to everything that it can perceive in the visual field placed before it. Everything. So, to see like a mirror, we will want to both feel and see with the entire body and to view the entire field as a unified field, not focusing on some aspects of it while excluding others.

Can you let yourself see everything at once without focusing on anything in particular? When you open your vision to reflect the whole of the visual field, the field of vision appears roughly elliptical and bends around you slightly on each side, like wraparound sunglasses.* Let yourself be as aware of the peripheries of the visual field—way off on the right and left sides, way up at the top as well as at the bottom—as you are of

---

*If you close one eye, the visual field looks approximately circular, but when you look with both your eyes, the visual field looks decidedly elliptical. To compose a circle, after all, you need a single center point, but to compose an ellipse, you need two centers.

any central feature in it. Let yourself see how vision fades at its peripheries into areas beyond your field of sight.

The hawk looks with laserlike precision, searching the meadow beneath for a rodent to munch on. For the purposes of Shenxiu's poem, though, let go of looking for anything in particular or focusing your visual awareness on just one object in the visual field. Let yourself see everything. And let yourself feel everything while you're doing that.

Paying such global attention to the visual field depletes thoughts' soil, leaving them no place to take root. Veils of thought only appear as you lose awareness of what's in front of you to be seen and inside of you to be felt.

When you're lost in thought, you diminish your visual acuity and lose sight of the visual field. A dusty layer of thought, like a drawn curtain, comes between you and what you're looking at, and so the visual field recedes and separates itself from you.

But if you awaken body and open fully to vision, the internal monologue starts fading from inside your head. What replaces the fading parade of thoughts? The visual field replaces it. You can actually feel the visual field penetrating into the physical space in the middle of your head that unbidden thought ordinarily occupies and fills. And when this happens, you begin to melt into a merged union with what you ordinarily perceive to exist so separate from, and outside of, yourself.

When mind becomes a mirror, the conscious perception of vision replaces the unconscious ramblings of thought. At first, the emerging awareness of body starts melting the monologue. Then vision comes in to wipe the slate of the monologue clean, like a schoolchild erasing sentences off a blackboard.

Before we move forward and start exploring different techniques and meditations that help correlate body, vision, and mind into a unified, coterminous phenomenon, take a moment and reverse the direction of your looking. Don't be so concerned about what you're looking out on, but try instead to locate where exactly it is you're looking from.

Lost in thought, the place from which you look is centered in your anatomical eyes, but when thought lifts, you don't just look from the locus of your eyes anymore, do you? Don't you look from a place somewhere behind your eyes, inside your head, down even into your body?

Where is it that you look from? Answering this question is not a simple task because as you keep looking for the place you're looking from, that place keeps morphing, drawing you ever deeper into your body, into yourself. Keep going deeper. Keep looking for the place you look from (clue: it's deep inside you and isn't just the place from which you see; it's also the place where you are). If you can let the whole of the visual field merge and mate with this place you're looking from, joining the two as lovers in a tryst, you may suddenly find yourself somewhere far behind your eyes, but not feeling separated at all from the world you look out on (can the surface of a mirror ever be separated from the images reflected onto it?).

Hui Neng tells us to look directly inside at the nature of the mind. Shenxiu tells us that the nature of the mind is closely tied to an alliance of awakened body and clear perception. Right behind your eyes, you are there. Can you find yourself there? Can you find where you are? Can you keep locating the place inside your head where you're looking from? What if the place you're looking from is what you're looking for?

THREE

Through the Looking Glass

*at all times we must work to keep it polished
and not let any dust collect*

When we first sit down to meditate, we're often instructed to close our eyes, to shut out the world outside ourselves over which we so incessantly obsess, and focus instead on the world inside ourselves, which we so often overlook. Ordinarily we're so fixated on the objects and events in the world we look out on, the world *out there,* that we tend to forget about the parallel universe that exists *in here,* inside ourselves, inside our body and mind. So we shut our eyes . . . and the world inside starts to appear in the form of sensations and energies in the body and thoughts and images in the mind.

That a world exists inside our body and mind—a world just as vast and mysterious, fascinating and complex, as pleasurable and painful as the world outside our body and mind—is one of the revelations of meditating with closed eyes. When we close our eyes, the distractions of the world temporarily disappear, and it's easier to perceive what's going on inside ourselves—our thoughts, feelings, hopes and fears, our sensations. Disengaging, if even for a few moments, from the sensory

39

overload of our modern world, we enter into a private world that we alone have access to.

But the pendulum of awareness was never meant to stay stuck in its focus on the interior world of thoughts, feelings, and sensations any more than on the exterior world of visual objects. Once we become more conversant with our inner bodily world of sensation and thought, we can then reopen our eyes and view the world outside the body in a way that embraces both, not favoring one over the other. As vital as it is for those of us on a meditative path to explore and understand the workings of our inner life, it is equally important that we then marry the two—our inner and outer worlds—so we can expose and dissolve the dualistic bias that separates inner from outer, what Albert Einstein so aptly referred to as the optical delusion of consciousness.

With eyes open, you run the risk of getting so drawn out into the world you look out at that you forget yourself. With eyes closed, you run the risk of implosion, of becoming so drawn into your interior world that you bring compressed tension into the cranium, especially the area of the face surrounding the eyes. Establishing a mind that functions like a mirror allows you to partake of both worlds simultaneously without losing sight of either. The inner ground of awareness merges with the outer world you look on just as the surface of a mirror merges with the reflections of whatever's placed before it.

Each of the meditations in this chapter presents a different strategy for dissolving distorting layers of accumulated thought residue and keeping the mirror of the mind as clear as possible. As you explore them, remember to pay equal and simultaneous attention to both the world you look out on and the place inside your head from which you look. By engaging both at once, you negate the possibility of getting caught up in either one at the expense of the other.

Meditations for Merging Body and Vision

Calibrating the Lens

The instruction to *keep it polished and not let any dust collect* is addressed as much to the body as to the mind. Body is the foundational ground of the mirror, so you always want to tend to it first.

As much as possible . . .

Keep the body shining and sparkling through remembering to open to feeling presence. Do your best not to let any unnecessary tension distort the clear shimmer of the body through inviting unnecessary holding, frozen stillness, and lack of resilience into its tissues. Do your best not to let any dust accumulate on the clear mirror of the mind through becoming lost in thought forms that are themselves dependent on, and coemergent with, tensions in the body. Keep cleaning off the residues of tension and contraction that have accumulated in the body and mind through remembering to let go, relax, softening into felt presence.

To create a visual lens whose calibration allows us to view the world through a mind like a mirror, body first needs to be deeply relaxed and fully felt. Tensions in the body serve to numb the body's sensations, effectively putting it to sleep.

Tensions in the body create the kinds of mirrors that you find in amusement parks whose warps and irregularities create distortions in their reflections, so you may be able to see yourself as a tall, elegant dancer or a squat, disfigured gnome, rather than as you are. Tension anywhere in the body eventually spreads and works its way through the entire body, robbing body of its relaxation and seeding the mind with unbidden thought.

The first and most important step in calibrating this lens is just to let yourself feel. Every little part. All at once. Everything. When you can relax into feeling everything all at once, vision opens naturally.

The fundamental practice is simply this: let yourself feel, and then let yourself see.

❧ Single Vision

> *the eye is the lamp of the body*
> *let your eye be single*
> *and the whole body will be filled with light*
> LUKE 11:34

The visual field may be of one piece, but still we have two eyes with which to view it. The binocularity of our vision gives us a perception of depth that a single eye can't provide, but it also exposes us to the possibility that our eyes will function independently of each other and remain out of sync. Just as we're right- or left-handed, most of us favor viewing the world through one of our eyes over the other, and this ocular dominance causes the energies in the middle of the cranium, at the eye center, to become imbalanced and, effectively, to split in two. When the energies of the eyes are imbalanced in this way, like two gears that don't mesh, mind tends to split in two as well, forfeiting its felt sense of integration and going off into different thought forms and personas behind each eye. When each eye and side of the brain is in a kind of competition for the energies at our eye center, we tend to stay locked in thought.

Integrating and inviting back into balance the energies in both the right and left eyes, so that they start intermingling with each other rather than repelling each other, lets us start looking out at the world from the vantage of single, instead of bifurcated, vision. When we see with single vision, the visual field starts appearing as a unified field whose location in space is not so much *out there* anymore as right *in here* in the middle of our cranium, and unbidden thought forms to the right or the left recede. As thought recedes, body lights up. It bursts into sensation, just as Jesus suggests.

Begin this meditation by paying attention to the feeling presence in each of your eyes separately. Start by placing your awareness in your left eye, as well as the space behind the eye. Center yourself entirely in the left side of your head, behind your left eye, almost as though you were a creature with only one eye. If it helps, you can cover your right eye with your right hand.

Feel the presence and sensation in your eye and in the space behind your eye, in the whole left side of your cranium, and watch what starts happening both to your vision and sense of self. Spend several minutes examining what it feels like to be completely focused in your left eye alone and how this affects what the world looks like. Keep relaxing into the feeling space in your cranium behind your eye. Who are you when you become the person who sees solely through your left eye?

Now reverse sides. Move your awareness over into your

right eye and your right-sided vision. It may take some time to make the transition over, so be patient; gradually, the feeling presence in your right eye will emerge (once again, it may be helpful to cover your left eye with your left hand). What can you feel behind this eye? Does it feel different from what you felt behind your left eye? Who are you when you let your right-eyed vision become dominant?

What kinds of thoughts and self-images come to you when you put your entire attention into each of your eyes, withdrawing attention from the other? Does the visual field look different? Does your sense of self feel different? Is one side naturally more receptive, the other more engaging?

Now . . . let yourself feel both eyes simultaneously.

When you first feel both eyes at once, each eye will feel like a distinct and separate energetic entity, orbiting around its own center of gravity, out of sync with and repelling the other. Slowly, let the dissonant sensations and energies in each of your eyes (and in the space behind your eyes) start to relax and intermingle, feeling each other out, right exploring left, left exploring right, coming together and mixing rather than staying so apart and separate. You can't force this merger to occur. You can't, and wouldn't want to, try to make one of your eyes feel more like the other. You just want to relax and let go, allowing the surface tensions to soften and subside organically, on their own, so that the feeling presence of vision can become more unified.

To allow the bifurcated energies in your eyes to relax and blend, you have to let go of seeing from your anatomical eyes and move backward behind your eyes, behind the energetic barrier of dissonance, back inside your cranium, even perhaps down into the back of the body itself. Just keep experimenting as you make your way back to a place, deep within the cranium, that allows the energies in the eyeballs and their surrounding orbits to relax into each other, letting you suddenly see from a perspective of single vision. In this way, the feeling presence in the pineal gland, which esoteric philosophers point to as the seat of higher vision, naturally becomes more activated.

See as with one eye, not two. Feel the relaxation at the surface of your face, the dissolving of the persona that you wear like a mask, the merging of the two separate eye energies into a single lens of vision. The key to knowing that you've found your way into single vision is that your body will start to wake up, to tingle and make its presence felt. Who do you become when you follow Jesus's suggestion to see with single vision and light up your body?

Eyes of the Head, the Heart, the Belly

When the feeling presence at your eye center splits in two, you stay locked in your eyes and head, and unbidden thought proliferates. Seeing solely with the eyes of your head, you bring tension into the cranium and reinforce your perception of separation between your inner and outer worlds.

But when you start relaxing the tensions in your physical eyes, the two centers from which you look come together as a more unified presence and coalesce in a single location somewhere in back of your physical eyes. When you can relax so deeply that the place from which you see moves from the surface of your physical eyes into the area of the back of your neck, down even into the middle of your upper torso, you start seeing through the eyes of the heart. Unbidden thought starts turning itself off, and it's easier to feel more unified in yourself and in your relationship with the world you look out on as well.

And if you keep relaxing the eyes and the body even more, you can feel your locus of vision drop down even farther, deep into your belly. When your belly becomes the place from which you see, you enter into an even greater dissolve, where you and the world you look out on may feel even more conjoined.

So . . . put yourself in your eyes. Let yourself be the person who sees from your eyes and is out of touch with the feeling presence behind your eyes. Become the person who solely sees with and through the eyes of your head. Whom do you become when you look out from your eyes alone, and what kind of world do you see?

Next, move your awareness back and down, behind your eyes. Let yourself see from the feeling presence in the back of your neck and upper back. Let the awakened feeling presence in this part of your body become the center from which you see. See how the tensions in the eyes relax as you do this. See how your perspective on the world you look out on starts to shift as you feel more empathically related to the visual field. Awaken the feeling presence in the middle of your chest, and integrate that feeling presence with your seeing. Whom do you become when you start centering yourself in, and seeing through, the eyes of the heart?

And then drop down and relax even further. Let your completely relaxed belly and lower back become the pupil of your eye and the center of your vision. Grounding yourself in the feeling presence in the belly, seeing from its felt center, lets you dissolve right into and through visual field, and when visual field shows up so dramatically, thought vanishes.

From the eyes, you move back and down into your heart lens. Out of your heart, you drop down even farther into your belly. Seeing through the eyes of the head keeps you fixated on the outer world. Seeing through the eyes of the heart keeps you and the world you look out on in more equitable balance. Seeing though the eyes of the belly keeps you probing depths of soul and the great ground of being.

Front and Back

Imagine for a moment that you could divide your body in two, separating your front from your back. Everything to the front of this imaginary plane of division exists in one sphere of experience while everything to the back of this plane falls into another.

Place your awareness entirely in your front sphere, and start by taking inventory of everything your front consists of. In terms of your physical body, there are sensations radiating outward through its surface as well as a mind that can only view the world through the frontal eyes of the head. This quality of mind creates a persona or mask that it dons as a mediating buffer between itself and the world. This mask, like all masks, sits right at the front of the body and creates the self-image you hope to portray to the world.

What else exists out at the front of the body? Our perception of the visual field exists there. The visual field is always and only in front of us, never behind, but mostly we view it as something *out there,* separate from us. Let yourself, for a moment, feel the front of everything as an integrated unit of experience—the sensations at the front of your body, your self-images and thoughts, the visual field itself, all three as integral component parts of your front.

Now shift your awareness to your back and to everything behind this imaginary plane of division. The back of your body houses and protects your spinal cord through which all nervous impulse passes. The back of the body, felt into as a unit completely separate from the front, is poor in thought, but rich in nervous impulse and reveals an invisible world of energies, sensations, and dimensions of consciousness just as real and, in its own way, vast as the frontal world of visual appearances. Just as the visual field in front of you goes on forever outward into the distance, so too can the invisible world in back of you be felt to go on, apparently forever, backward into the distant dark. Front and back reveal two different but complementary worlds, two different perspectives reflecting two different aspects of experience.

Explore them both, one at a time—your front as an integrated unit of sensation, persona, and visual field; your back as an integrated unit of sensation, silence, and interior universe.

What now happens when you remove the dissecting plane and experience the vastnesses of both worlds, front and back, simultaneously?

Seeing Wide

Mostly we view the world as a composite collection of individual, discrete objects, but the dimension of experience that Rumi refers to as union, in which the common ground from which everything springs is directly felt and even seen, remains mostly invisible. To survive in this world, we learn to be highly selective in our vision, narrowly focusing on one primary object in the visual field over all the rest, seeing one thing at a time while ignoring everything else, almost as if we were passing a magnifying glass across the field of vision, and whatever appears before the glass pops out while everything beyond the glass fades and recedes.

Alternatively, though, we can learn to soften our eyes and widen our gaze, to see everything at once as a unified visual field without focusing in on anything in particular. To shift our vision from narrow to wide, we'll want to start paying as much attention to what's happening at the peripheries of the visual field as at its center. When we see wide in this way, just looking without looking at or for anything, we may lose our ability to distinguish one object from another, but the invisible world of union starts coming into felt focus.

Take a moment and let yourself look at any object across the room from where you're sitting. It doesn't matter what you select. It can be anything. Start narrowing your focus as much as possible on this one object, burning your gaze right into it, so that the object appears with intense clarity, but everything around it looks a bit blurry. Feel how one-pointed your mind becomes, but also how you have to bring tension and holding into your eyes to narrow your focus so intensely in this way.

And then let your vision go wide. Without losing your visual grounding with the object in the center of your vision, widen your gaze so that you can also see what's way off to either side of your roughly elliptical visual field. See how the definitions in the objects at the peripheries of your vision, far to the right and left, start fading into the space outside your visual field. Fixing your gaze on an object in the center of your visual field, while simultaneously remaining aware of what exists way off to your right and left, shifts your locus of vision toward the back of the head and relaxes tension in the eyes, neck, chest, and back, and eventually through the whole of the body.

If you then add whatever appears to you at the top and bottom margins of your visual field as well, the whole of the visual field will present itself in the form of a mandala, an image of wholeness and unity.

Start by focusing on anything. Then go wide and include everything. See it all at once, the center of your world as well as its edges.

Inviting Vision

Because we so view the visual field as existing *out there,* our eyes mostly reach out and grab at its objects. Reaching out with our vision, however, brings tension to the eye center and projections and interpretations to the mind. It also keeps us locked within the perception of separation as the sole perspective from which reality can be profitably viewed.

See what happens when you consciously reverse this polarity, so that you no longer reach out at the visual field—through the ocular equivalent of outstretched arms—but invite it to come to you instead. Offer this invitation wholeheartedly, without any reservations, and watch how the visual field starts to penetrate and project itself right into you, eventually taking up residence in the space where thoughts would otherwise reside. Discover what it is that you have to do in your body and mind to issue this invitation (the visual field will always graciously accept).

Inviting the visual field to step forward in this way and

enter right into you, allowing it to mate with, and imprint itself on, the clear mirror of the mind, washes away obscuring residues of thought dust in a sudden, dramatic flash, as though you've taken a hose to the windshield of a car that's just been driven across a dusty desert. Through this welcoming gesture of invitation, the visual field itself becomes the agent that cleanses your perception of it.

Grounding through Vision

At times, as body awakens, strong sensations and energies may be released and felt to sweep through you. At those moments, should they arise, it's even more important to stay grounded in vision. Always let sensations and energies emerge in your practices. Never hold back on them. So that you don't become overwhelmed, however, and feel that you have to brace yourself against what's happening in your body and mind, remember to look and see. Open to the visual field, welcome it in, and watch how it grounds you, even in the midst of strong, surging sensations, like a lightning rod in a storm.

One of the visual field's most helpful functions is to provide a grounding tether during episodes of powerful sensational swells, when the current of the life force causes your inner river of sensations to churn, like a spring stream into which too much winter runoff is pouring. Know that there's no need to hold back these floodwaters. Let them surge as they like. Just tie yourself to the visual field and pass through the flood. All floodwaters eventually recede.

Blowing the Dust Away

The act of polishing the mirror can be viewed as the conscious and intentional releasing and dissolving away of the barrier of unbidden thought and mental image, which in turn allows a more intimate joining together of the place from which you look and the objects you gaze out at. One of the most effective and powerful cleansing agents we have at our disposal, but that we often keep under literal wraps, is our breath.

When body is asleep, breath slumbers as well. But as body wakes up, so does breath. The tensions that put body to sleep also become roadblocks that stop breath in its tracks, not letting its natural transmitted motions make their way, joint by joint, through the body. As body awakens and as the wraps and held tension that keep breath constrained soften, breath naturally becomes fuller, more expansive in its inhalation, more complete in its exhalation.

To clean a mirror, we keep moving our cloth back and forth across its entire surface. To clean our body of its residues of tension and sleepiness, we can breathe in and out, consciously, intentionally, feeling how breath can be felt to touch into every place in the body, stimulating sensation everywhere as it passes through, not unlike how a wave moves through a body of water. Just as your polishing cloth needs to rub every square inch of the surface of the mirror you're cleaning, so does the breath want to touch into, and stimulate sensation on, every little part of the body, over and over and over again.

So let yourself breathe . . . and feel the whole of the body.

Let yourself breathe . . . and open to the whole of the visual field.

At those moments when you breathe into the whole body, leaving no little felt part out, while simultaneously breathing into the whole of the visual field, leaving no little visual part out, thought crumbles, and behind the crumbling edifice essential nature is revealed.

Let breath be a cloth and cleaning agent to awaken sensation throughout the body and dissolve the layer of thought that covers over the mind like dust and grime on a mirror's surface. In this way, every breath you take can become an agent of cleansing and healing.

As Rumi says,

> *bringing breath to life*
> *is the essence of every religion*
> *and the remedy for every illness*
> *let every breath you take*
> *cleanse the soul of its grief and pain*
> *so it can keep glowing brightly inside you*

The Three Levels of Vision

The great Buddhist teacher Bodhidharma is said to have sat in front of a wall, with open eyes, for several years before healing the separation between inner and outer and attaining the awakened state. For this exercise, sit down a few feet away from a wall in upright meditation posture.

Open your eyes and let yourself look directly at the wall. Begin by just gazing at the physical wall in front of you in the most conventional way, as an individuated entity separate from the wall you're looking out at—you sitting here, the wall in front of you there. As soon as you start gazing at the wall, you enter into felt relationship with it, but at this level of vision there are distinct boundaries and demarcations between you and the wall, between you as observer and the wall as observed. This first level of vision is the one most familiar to us. It's how we customarily look and see, and it reflects our belief in how reality is constructed—that the wall and I are separate events, destined never to intermingle, never to coalesce. This level of vision views objects as solid and dense, each existing in its own little exclusive pocket of physical space. From this most common sense of perspectives, two objects can never occupy the same position in space, and *touch* can only be felt to occur through the physical contact of hand and wall.

To initiate the second level of vision, gradually let body start coming awake. Over a period of several minutes, welcome feeling presence back into awareness, relaxing and softening tensions as you bring the sensations of the body back to felt life. As feeling presence comes forward, body starts experiencing itself directly, not as solid object, but as felt field of shimmering, minute, vibratory sensations and energies. And now, as you're able to feel body more and more as river of sensations, watch what starts happening to the appearance of the wall in front of you.

When you hold back on surrendering into felt presence, the wall—or any object you turn your gaze to—appears solid, its surface hard and opaque. But when you bring body to life, when you awaken it and enter the shimmer, a remarkable thing starts occurring. The surface of the wall starts lightly shimmering as well. Sometimes the wall's shimmer may look like millions of tiny little lights flickering on and off. Sometimes it may more closely resemble the appearance of heat waves viewed across a desert floor, and no, you're not hallucinating. You're simply seeing what the wall looks like when viewed through the eyes of a body that's awakened its felt presence. Ask yourself honestly—is not the surface of the wall percolating, bristling with energy, alive in subtle movements and shimmer, not unlike the felt body that's looking at it? Ours is a magical world, but we have to soften the patterns of tension and holding and awaken the body to its shimmer before we can see it so.

Finally, as you keep relaxing and surrendering even further, you may find yourself dropping down into a third level of vision in which the shimmer of both body and wall start magnetically to reach out to each other, like partners in a dance, responding to the other's motions, strangely commingling, and eventually merging back together into a coterminous, shared dimension of experience. Not unlike Alice falling through the rabbit hole, you may suddenly feel yourself disappearing right into and through the wall you're gazing at, as though vision has led you to the felt perception of an alternate reality, a substratum or ground state permeating the world of the ten thousand objects, but somehow binding all of them together in a piece. When you and the wall start interacting in such a deep and intimate way, what happens to *you?* Where do *you* go?

Starting off from a place of little felt awareness and a perception of separation, you enter the shimmer—of both you and the world—and then you fall even further into a place at which, if even just for a little minute, you merge with whatever it is you're looking out on.

Body, Vision, and Sound

A valid criticism of the singular tack I have chosen for this book to sail on is that every sensory field, not just the field of vision, can be related to with mirrorlike clarity (or provide you with ample sensory input for interpretation, projection, and reaction). What, for example, of sound? While smell and taste may arguably be considered of lesser importance in the establishment of a clear vision of reality, sound is as omnipresently vital an expression of the sensorium as is vision.

While the visual field enters us through the eyes at the front of the face and the invisible world can be felt to extend back behind us, sound enters us from the side, through our right and left ears, and provides ballast and balance to the merger of body and vision. Sound is like the horizontal bar that a tightrope walker uses to maintain balance as he or she walks along a slender cord strung between the rooftops of two buildings. Sound grounds and sanctifies the marriage of body and vision.

If you look upon sensation, sound, and vision as the angles of a triangle, watch what happens when you create a perfect equilaterality between them. Be as aware of sensations as you are of vision as you are of sound. Opening to, and balancing out, an awareness of these three primary fields grounds you in the dimension of mirrorlike mind. When body, vision, and sound are all simultaneously experienced as whole fields, errant thought simply falls away; the fields themselves start, strangely, to merge with one another; and you find yourself vanishing right through this commingled awareness into the dimension of essential nature.

So . . . let yourself listen. To everything that you can hear. Not just the pleasant sounds. Not just to the voice that's speaking to you, but to everything—the background murmur of the room in which you sit, the barrage of random noise of the modern city soundscape, the nurturing sounds of nature, the sounds inside your own body.

Now add vision. See the whole of the visual field as a unified field, everything all at once. And then complete the triangle of awareness by adding sensation, relaxing into and feeling the entire body all at once.

Never strive to experience something special. It's just about opening to what's here before you. This sound. This vision. This sensation. Just this.

A monk once asked the Zen master Joshu for a secret teaching, "What is the word of the ancients?" Joshu simply replied, "Listen carefully! Listen carefully!"

In a similar vein, the Greek author Nikos Kazantzakis once asked a monk, "When will my turn come to see God?"

"It's easy, very easy," he answered. "Just open your eyes and you'll see Him."

Never strive to feel, see, or hear anything special. *Just this* is the secret doorway.

Blinking

Most of us blink many times a minute as a way to keep the surface of the eyeballs moist and free of irritants and the lens of vision as clean and unobstructed as possible (not unlike how we spritz the windshield of a moving car with a liquid solution as we hit the wiper button to make sure that the windshield remains clear and unobstructed). In addition to this reflexive physiological function, however, there exists a wholly other intentional psychological function to the action of blinking.

When thought forms coalesce in the space behind the eyes, they create an encasing, energetic barrier, a solid wall that keeps the naturally expansive presence of embodied consciousness contained and collapses our sense of self into the space in the center of our cranium. This contraction of presence promotes our belief in the irreconcilable separation between what we call *inner* and *outer*. It encases us inside a kind of energetic shrink-wrap and distorts what we see.

Melting that contractive barrier has been the main theme of this book, and we have offered a number of strategies for effecting that change. A further simple strategy is the intentional, repetitive blinking of the eyes.

Blinking the eyes, rapidly in succession, has the effect of popping the encasing energetic balloon inside of which unbidden thought so successfully encloses us. Blinking the eyes repetitively emits a laserlike burst of energy that disintegrates the restricting barrier, helping thought to dissolve and presence to expand outward once again, embracing and merging with the visual field as the barrier melts away.

When you find yourself obsessively lost in thought, remember to blink your eyes in rapid succession. Thought disappears, presence expands, and you settle back down into the clarity of essential nature.

Building on the earlier explorations to awaken the body, the preceding meditations can lead you directly to the embodied and altogether natural consciousness in which mind behaves as mirror, not as interpreter, not as projector. This dimension of experience, in which the optical delusion of separation is revealed not to be the sole perspective from which the world can be viewed, is a birthright state for all of us as we continue to ride the great current of the life force and evolve as a species. Experiencing the merging of the place from which you look and that out on which you look melts and heals pain and tension in the body and opens mind to its most essential nature. It also simply feels right, like coming back home after a long and perhaps arduous time away.

Keep refining and exploring vision. Keep paying attention to what you can see and how things appear. The following supplemental exercises may help expand your ability to look and see. The more you look and the more you see, the more mind has no choice but to start functioning more like a mirror.

◥◉◜ What Color Is It?

One of my best friends from university days is an artist. For many years he traveled the world, a pack of clothing and paints on his back, not wanting to settle down anywhere. As he said, "Everywhere you go has a different quality of light and color," and he didn't want to confine himself to any one palette. In those days it was easy to lose track of him, as he would spend long months in Montana and then suddenly pick up and move down to Haiti, only to show up in Arizona several years later.

Oftentimes, when we were together, we enjoyed playing the What Color Is It? game. We would sit next to each other and look out over an expansive landscape—trees, mountains, water, clouds, the sun and its reflected light. After a few minutes, one of us might turn to the other and say, "Look over there, at the top of that tree. If you were to paint that as accurately as possible, what colors would you use to paint the top of the tree?" Or the clouds. Or the mountains. Or the waves on the water.

Ordinarily we think of the sky as blue and trees as green and leave it at that. But when we really let ourselves look with a discerning eye, we often find that there are a multitude of different, subtle shadings and tones in any object that we look at. The sky is rarely just blue. There are hues of grays and whites and a hundred different tones, shades, and tints of blue, maybe even a trace, depending on the time of day, of lavenders, greens, and corals (and lavenders, greens, and corals can have hundreds of different tones, shades, and tints). Trees aren't just green. They're every conceivable shade in the stable of green, and we haven't even started looking at the branches and the trunk (They're hardly just *brown*, are they?).

Play this game with a friend if you like; no winners or losers, just each of you offering your observations. Be as precise as you can in your discernments and color pronouncements, like the visual equivalents of wine connoisseurs who somehow recognize the tastes of wines to be like ripe loganberry, mocha, or truffles. To forge a common vocabulary of color, you may want to go into an art supply store and get a color chart with the traditional names of all the acrylic and oil-based paints.

This game takes time to settle into. The longer you look, the more subtleties you see. Ordinarily we're in too much of a hurry in our lives to notice the full, rich palette of the visual field, so it's helpful to remember to slow down, to stop and see the roses. What color are the roses? What color are the stems and leaves and the surrounding ground? What colors do you use to paint a night sky of dappled clouds with reflected light from the moon?

Cloud Gazing

Speaking of clouds, some of us have been fortunate enough to have special memories of lying on our backs on the ground as small children, carefree, looking up at the sky, and letting our imagination roam as a parade of puppy dogs, dragons, armies, and angels kept emerging through the clouds. Faces and shapes—some beautiful, some spooky—would appear out of nowhere, act out an archetypal drama in front of our eyes, disperse with the wind, and then change into something altogether different. Ah, the joys of pretechnological childhood!

Cloud gazing can be a powerful tool, in this case not to see things as they are but, as Anaïs Nin earlier suggested, to see things as we are. In the clouds I see myself. In the clouds I project the issues that so occupy me. Like the famous inkblot tests, in which one person may see a demon and another a saint, the drama acted out in the clouds is a pure projection of your deep, unconscious mind. Many of your cloud visions will resonate with the image you mostly hold of yourself. Others may confound or even disturb you. No matter. Just look and see what appears.

This meditation is best done on a relatively warm and somewhat blustery day. Lying on your back, just start watching the clouds. Don't try to make anything appear. Just look and wait and see. And when something does appear, welcome it into your vision, and then watch how it changes its shape, turns into something completely different, or disperses altogether into space.

Even briskly moving clouds move at a pace far slower than the clip of culture. Lying on your back, gazing up at the clouds, you can let the hectic rush of city life go and start resonating with a much slower pulse of motion. Every time you lie on your back and gaze up at the clouds, you watch a minidrama unfold. Every time you lie and gaze, you cocreate a new short story. Link the appearances together and turn them into a narrative. Kittens become candles. Serpents become princes. Maybe, over the course of ten minutes of gazing, you'll see three distinct images. Like a three-card tarot spread, what story are they telling you?

Sky Gazing

And then what happens when the clouds disperse and the sky is an expanse of blue? Not a cloud anywhere to be seen. Just open, empty sky. Deep blue. Penetrating blue.

Just as you looked at the wall a few exercises ago, just as you look at the changing shapes of clouds, let yourself look and gaze out into the infinity of a cloudless sky. Nothing to meet you. Nothing to interact with. Just a deep empty space that you can relax into completely and keep falling into forever.

A deep blue sky lets you pour yourself into it. It not only invites and welcomes you to expand into it, it behaves like a vacuum, actually sucking you into its vastness. Let go and dissolve into that vastness. Become the infinite emptiness of the cloudless sky. On every exhalation, feel yourself dissolving away into and through the portal of the sky. On every inhalation, feel the vastness of the sky enter back into you.

The greater the expanse of clear sky, the easier it is to explore this meditation from the Tibetan tradition. On the top of a mountain, on a boat far out at sea, driving across a great plain, the sky is a dominating presence, a colossus, hovering over everything. Sit in upright meditation posture. Gaze at the sky. Feel how the sky is tugging at you. Surrender to its pull. Where is it taking you?

Kasinas

During the time of the Buddha, small disks of different colors were used as objects of concentration for the meditator to gaze at. Meditators would sit down in upright sitting posture and focus their entire attention on the colored shape, the *kasina,* that was pinned to a wall at eye level, right in front of them, just a few feet away. Meditating on a kasina helps focus the mind, balance out the right and left energies at the eye center, and develop strong, but relaxed, concentration. It also supports the direct awakening of bodily sensation, as it's difficult to focus on a kasina without almost immediately becoming more aware of bodily presence.

The kasina that's illustrated on the final page of the book adds a dimension of contrasting colors to accentuate the effect even further. With this or any kasina, simply sit down and start gazing at it. Start by focusing on the colored dot in the center of the triangle, and then gradually expand your vision so you're seeing not only the center dot but the whole of the kasina as well.

As you do this, the colors and shapes will start to morph and even merge at times in a dazzling optical display. Just sit and look and allow. Colors shift and shift back. Forms merge and separate. Edges of colors bleed into each other only to again become sharply defined. Don't try to hold on to any appearance. Just let go through vision and watch the shifting display.

Sitting with a kasina takes you on a progressive journey down through each of the three levels of vision. Starting out from a place of you and the kasina, it doesn't take long before both your body and the kasina start shimmering and you begin to merge with and through it. Layer after layer, level after level, watch how your perception of both the kasina and your own body and mind keeps changing and shifting. In this way, you become more aware of how the current of the life force flows through both you and the visual field, surging here, subsiding there, always on the move.

The kasina's veil-dropping dance and light show can start quickly, sometimes within the first few seconds of meditation. So long as you keep relaxing, not resisting the visual shifts and optical play, not grabbing on to any one appearance or holding anything back either, the dance will continue, on and on.

When you're finished with a session of kasina gazing (it can go on for as little as a minute or two or be extended indefinitely), shut your eyes and focus on the afterimage that starts appearing behind your closed lids. The shape of the afterimage is identical to the kasina, but its colors will be the exact opposite of the colors of the kasina you've been gazing at.

Sometimes the afterimage of a kasina can be even more visually impactful than the kasina itself. Let yourself watch and delight in this afterimage until it fades completely away.

Eye Gazing

All the little meditations that have been presented here so far are solo excursions that you alone can take and explore. For this meditation, however, you'll need a partner.

While everyone's spiritual journey is theirs and theirs alone to take, still we are social creatures in constant interaction with others. It's challenging enough, on your own, to awaken the body and explore the quality of mind that functions more like a mirror. It becomes even more challenging to do this in the company of others with whom you're directly conversing or interacting.

Gazing at the wall in front of you, the clouds above you, or a kasina placed before you is a private, intimate act. But what happens when you turn your gaze away from the wall, the clouds, the sky, the kasina and look directly into the eyes of your friend? Ours is a culture suspicious of the energies of an awakened body, and holding the gaze of a friend almost immediately awakens strong sensations and energies in the body. The primary reason we so rarely engage others in direct eye contact is that we've become so accustomed to a consciousness in which we've lost awareness of sensation and become consumed in thought that this sudden surge of feeling presence, like an electrical jolt that passes through both you and your friend, can be startling. However, if you can both welcome this sudden surge of sensation and keep relaxing into it, then the practice can take you into a fascinating and completely natural condition of body and mind that is difficult to access so easily any other way.

When you and your friend sit across from each other, holding the other's gaze, the first thing you may become aware of are rumblings of awakening through your bodies. Some of these rumblings may be very pleasurable. Others may make you feel decidedly uncomfortable as the practice forces you to feel what's actually going on in your body at this moment of time. If you can relax into the intensified sensations that the practice catalyzes, accepting them as they are, allowing them to shift and change organically, on their own, at their own pace, then the practice starts deepening. Both you and your friend may find your bodies starting strongly to shimmer, and at this point the visual field may start to alter its appearance in a most dramatic fashion.

The hard edges of your friend's face may soften. You may start seeing a glow or even colors surrounding his or her face and body. The image of your friend's face may darken or lighten unexpectedly. At times your friend's face may disappear, only to dissolve into effulgent light, only to reappear a moment later. Your friend's face may even take on a whole different appearance and look like someone you've never known or met. Just as sensations keep shifting, so too does the show of visual appearances keep morphing right in front of you.

And finally, you may enter an even deeper level of the gaze where you and your friend no longer feel like such separate, individuated entities, but rather somehow connected and joined together into a single, shared expression of being—of soul. The practice couldn't be simpler really. You and your friend sit down across from each other, turn your eyes toward each other, hold the gaze, and then just let go and surrender to the ride of shifting sensation and vision. So simple a practice, and yet so challenging and often fearful for humans to engage in.

You don't need a teacher or even someone familiar with the practice to open it for you. This isn't the kind of practice that you need to attend a special school or training to study and learn. All you need is your friend. Sit down together, open your eyes, hold each other's gaze, and trust in whatever happens next, and in whatever happens after that. Keep relaxing into the contact and lose yourself in the gaze.

Mirror Gazing

To prepare yourself for entering into the gaze with your friend, you may first want to spend some time with a kasina or gazing at your own reflection in a mirror. Both of those practices kindle many of the same kinds of effects—melting tension, dissolving barriers, entering into a shimmering union with the object of your gaze—as does gazing into the eyes of your friend. For some people, the practice of gazing with your friend feels the most powerful. For other people, doing sitting meditation practice in front of a kasina or a mirror feels more natural.

Sit down in upright meditation posture in front of a full-length mirror, and start gazing at your reflection in the mirror. Gaze right at and into your reflected eyes. What happens to you when you do this? What happens to your awareness of body, your awareness of mind? Just let go and allow sensations to break out—emerging, streaming, disappearing, reappearing, constantly changing. Just let go and let thoughts pass through and over, bubbling, flashing, perambulating, but never taking root. Holding your own gaze in a mirror while meditating grounds your felt sense of presence in the midst of the sometimes turbulent emergences and shiftings of body and mind.

What happens when you do your daily sitting practice in front of a mirror, just as Rumi suggests?

> *I came and brought you a mirror*
> *don't turn your face away*
> *look at yourself in the mirror, my child*

Seeing with the whole body reveals a different world from the one we conventionally live in. Even though we've presented the practice through the lens of Shenxiu's poem, there is nothing exclusively Buddhist about this practice. We all have eyes, we all have a body, and we all have a choice, no matter our background or religious orientation, to observe a world of separation or experience a world in which inner and outer are no longer at such odds with each other. Every activity you can engage in—whether you're formally sitting in meditation; walking in the mountains; pushing your buggy through a supermarket aisle; or praying in a church, a synagogue, or a mosque—presents you with this choice.

Adjusting the lens through which you look out on the world—from a setting in which the body is sleepy and the mind cloudy to an aperture in which the body has woken up and the mind is clear—can be as easy as snapping your fingers (abracadabra, behold the vision) or as challenging as getting a large ship, sailing along briskly in the open ocean, suddenly to change course and turn around 180 degrees. The ocular pattern of tension and holding that creates the first level of vision—in which we and what we look out on are forever perceived as separate, independent events—is deeply ingrained in all of us, and yet it can be relaxed.

Sometimes that reversal of direction is difficult to enact, like training a stubborn animal, and we have to keep reminding (and rebodying) ourselves over and over again to relax and melt the tensions that keep the second and third levels of vision unavailable. At other times, in an instant, it can be as simple as remembering to let the visual field come streaming into you, like a flash flood in a dry canyon, washing away the dusty you of pain and tension. Paying attention to vision, nurturing your relationship with the visual field, as though the visual field were your lover and bonded partner, allows moments of transformative vision in which there is very clearly far more going on than meets the eye.

These sudden moments of unexpected insight, moments that allow us to see the world in a whole different light, are often referred to as moments of epiphany (from the Greek *epi,* which means "highest," and *phanos,* which means "sight"). Through epiphany, this sudden seeing of things from a heightened perspective, we learn to see things as they are. Through his four simple lines of instruction, a miracle of pith and precision, Shenxiu offers us epiphany, a radical shift in how we ordinarily view ourselves and our world. What more could we ask for?

The epiphany is real, the description of the path elegant. Still, why did Shenxiu not win the contest? What about Hui Neng's four lines in response? What guidance do they offer, and why were they deemed more worthy of the prize?

AFTERWORD

The Monk Who Won
the Contest

But what of Hui Neng, the monk who won the contest and claimed the robe and bowl, the upstart who came from nowhere and undercut the monastery's favorite with his cheeky rebuttal? What of his poem? Clearly, something equally extraordinary can be found in its four naked lines, or the shocking outcome of the contest would certainly not have occurred.

> *there's really nothing like a tree of awakening*
> *nor is the mind anything at all like a mirror*
> *since everything is eternally empty of any*
> *   fundamental essence*
> *where could dust collect*

Let's be honest. Hui Neng's poem doesn't just express the truth of the dharma. It does it in a way that comes across as a slap to Shenxiu and, whether intentionally or not, delivers the message that its composer, and not Shenxiu, should be declared the winner of the contest and recognized as the dharma heir. Viewing the incident through a more contemporary lens, one might have wished that he could have done it in a way that was not such a direct and insulting repudiation of his fellow monk. More a fresh fruit than a dried one, any way you slice it, it's a juicy story—deception, betrayal, shock, a clash of visions, disappointment and elation, an extraordinary legacy for the ages. So what might the backstory to all of this be?

There are a number of conjectural possibilities (or conspiracy theories, if you like). It's certainly possible that Hui Neng was as genuinely guileless as he's first depicted during his initial interview with Hongren, a simple lad from the provinces who was fine with being assigned to kitchen duty and completely disinterested in monastery politics. Seeing Shenxiu's poem, he may have simply felt that it wasn't quite right and needed a little tweaking, innocently oblivious to the storm of repercussions his attempt at clarification was about to unleash. It's certainly a possibility.

As is the possibility that he wasn't so innocent and guileless after all, that perhaps after all the years on kitchen duty he may have been feeling slighted, on the short end of the stick of social bigotry held by people whose understanding of the dharma he may have viewed as far inferior to his own. Perhaps there had even been some enmity between him and Shenxiu in the past. Or . . . perhaps he harbored as much ambition, brilliantly concealed, as anyone tantalized by the prospect of winning a great prize. Perhaps.

On the other hand, it's possible that Hui Neng was not so simple of mind as is generally suggested, but not so Machiavellian either. Perhaps he simply didn't agree with Shenxiu's more pedestrian approach to practice, preferring attainment through a flashing moment of recognition rather than a long and slogging pilgrimage toward it. Perhaps he felt that the ineffable condition of essential nature can only be described in contrast to what it isn't, so the only way he could possibly express that truth was through negating Shenxiu's effort.*

Shenxiu was able to describe the whole of the path of practice, the terrain of approach, eloquently and simply, in just four short lines. In four equally short lines, Hui Neng conveyed the condition of arrival. In the end, though, are not path and goal equally necessary to complete each other? Are they not twins of a common heart, joined at the hip? Beyond that, does not Hui Neng require Shenxiu to express himself at all?

One of Hui Neng's legitimate concerns about Shenxiu's exposition may have been that it still supports the dualism of a self in here looking out on a world out there, that it posits the discovery of essential nature within the context of separation.

Shenxiu starts at the very beginning, with the observation that we're fractured in our awareness—body out of touch with feeling presence, feeling presence not integrated with mind, mind separated from the world it looks out on. From Shenxiu's perspective, not until the body is first awakened and mind starts functioning more like a mirror and less like an inter-

---

*An even more unsettling possibility, suggested by some scholars, is that the entire story of Shenxiu and Hui Neng was a fabrication, that neither of them actually existed, and that the contest was a clever public relations ploy on the part of subsequent schools of sudden enlightenment that wished to discredit the competing schools that spoke of a gradual ascent to the uncovering of essential nature. Do you think that a wisdom path as pure as the Buddhist dharma is above politics? Think again. However, even if the story of Shenxiu and Hui Neng is entirely allegorical (a supposition I personally doubt—why would someone from the sudden enlightenment school concoct a poem as remarkable as Shenxiu's if his purpose was to discredit him?), the perspectives that each of their poems represent are still directly applicable to those of us working to apprehend the core dimension of essential nature.

preter or projector, can we heal our misperceptions and find our way back to what Hongren viewed as essential nature.

Once that healing has occurred, though, even if only in a momentary flash of recognition, a new perspective is revealed from which it's now fair to say that there is no body, no mirror, no dust, only a universal ground dimension out from which all the individual objects of the world—all the things, all the bodies—emerge into form. Shenxiu talks about the relative, visible world that we've been born into. Hui Neng talks about the absolute, invisible—but equally palpable—perspective in which there's no longer so clear a distinction between inner and outer, body and world, body and mind, self and other.

Twenty-five hundred years ago, the Buddha instructed us to view the world as a dream or a bubble, a masterly illusion, a flashing show of appearances without anything like the underlying substantiality and sense of solidity we so readily ascribe to it. Today, quantum physicists echo this observation with their vision of a world in which the forces and building blocks that compose every object in the universe are constantly flashing in and out of existence. All matter, they further tell us, is mostly empty space.

Hindu cosmology, with which the Buddha would have been intimately familiar, also speaks of the world of appearances as an illusion, *maya,* a dream we mistake for reality, in contrast to the far more fundamental reality, *Brahman,* that underlies the show of appearances and out of which that show emerges.

The quantum physicist David Bohm, in the latter part of his life, came to the conclusion that our entire understanding of what constitutes reality needed a complete makeover and revamping. In a vision that directly reflects not only the

Buddha's words and the perspective of Hindu cosmology, but also the allegory of Plato's cave in which people misinterpret the dark shadows projected onto the walls of the cave as reality itself, he proposed that the world of appearances, what he calls the explicate order, is akin to a holographic light show that's being projected out from a mysterious, central source, which he refers to as the implicate order (and which, of course, religionists will be tempted to call God).

Why, Hui Neng might have mused, would you want to go to all the trouble of creating a mind like a mirror, a mind that's completely reflective of what's so illusory to begin with? Why not pass right through the world of appearances instead, right at the onset, in fact right now, and contact the source itself out of which all those appearances arise?

Just because it may be akin to a dream does not mean that you don't have to play scrupulously by its rules. But viewing appearances as a dream disrupts our conventional understanding of the nature of the world into which we've been born and allows the feeling presence of the body to break free of its self-imposed corral of confinement, radiating ever outward in a way that brings with it a physical comfort that feels like a birthright.

What if the Buddhists, Hindus, and quantum physicists are correct and the world of visual appearance is more virtual reality than actual reality? What if we've learned so effortlessly to navigate the explicate appearances of the virtual reality in which we live, like a clever gamer who may be more at home in the world perceived through the goggles he wears on his face, that we've completely forgotten that what we call reality may not be so substantively real after all? How gracefully can you glide through the world of appearances, projected as it may be from some mysterious central source, without losing your felt connection to that source?

It has always struck me as peculiar how we look at people and identify who they are with their very solid-looking face and body, but when we experience ourselves, we don't feel solid at all. Rather, we feel more like an empty, open space, infused with sensation and consciousness, hovering in and around and through the object of our physical body. From the outside looking in, everything looks so convincingly solid; from the inside feeling out, however, not nearly so much.

The Heart Sutra, one of Buddhism's most celebrated texts, tells us that there are two levels to everything we perceive. First, there's the very solid-looking, physical form—the book, the table, the tree, the person. Underlying this form, though, is a parallel dimension just as real and palpable as the solid-looking visual object, but essentially empty of anything that we conventionally call material substance. This substratum of emptiness is more like space than form, and the Heart Sutra, in equating the two as different manifestations of the same phenomena, makes it clear that everything partakes of both these dimensions.

If this notion of a sea of space and emptiness that underlies all form strikes you as too peculiar to seem credible, just remember your own body that looks so solid from the outside but feels so spacious from the inside. If this is so for your own body, why should this twofold expression of reality not be so for every other solid-looking physical object as well? So it's not just your body that partakes of this empty substratum, it's everything—the book, the table, the trees, the stars, the walls, anything at all that has visible form.

The most telling line of Hui Neng's poem, and the only one that is not a direct negation of Shenxiu, is "everything is eternally empty of any fundamental essence." For Hui Neng, the only thing that matters is a direct revelation of this dimension of emptiness underlying the form, so once again, he might ask, why focus on appearances, which is what a mind like a mirror must constantly do? Why not go straight away to the source, the core dimension of all things, the land where essential nature can immediately show its face?

Forms can be seen, but emptiness has to be felt. What happens when you make your way, level by level, down into your body? Initial numbness becomes a doorway to sensations; as sensations proliferate, they then become a direct link or conduit connecting and leading you to the substratum of emptiness that permeates all things. This formless dimension may be invisible to your eyes, but it's every bit as palpable as the book you hold in your hands. You can sense it here, everywhere, pulsing through your body.

What happens when you look out on the world and focus not on the appearance of the forms, but on the alternative field of emptiness that permeates all form? What happens when you pass right through the solid-looking appearance of the objects in your visual field to feel into, resonate with, and in a sense *see*, the parallel dimension of . . . emptiness?

This is Hui Neng's vision: don't get caught up in the distraction, no matter how fascinating it might appear; go straight to the fundamental source instead, right now, in this very moment.

In *Time, Space, and Knowledge* the Tibetan teacher Tarthang Tulku, in a sentiment perhaps stunning to ears so steeped in the legacy and ongoing inquiry of Western psychotherapy, has suggested that a primary source of all our frustrating mental and physical blocks and limitations is our belief that the surfaces of objects are opaque. What could he possibly mean by this?

If we only embrace the reality of the solid-looking form, but overlook and miss the parallel ground dimension of emptiness out of which all form emanates, surfaces of objects do indeed appear as opaque, impenetrable barriers that we can in no way breach or pass through. By focusing on only one-half of the stuff of reality, though, we end up fractured within ourselves and become ripe soil for neurosis to take root. By focusing only on the narrowness of form, we place an energetic straightjacket on ourselves, and this unnatural constraint causes painful pressures to build in the body and mind.

What he's getting at is that we play a kind of energetic but fictive game of bumper cars with what we conceive as solid objects in the visual field. When we awaken the body from its slumber of tension, we unleash a streaming phenomenon of shimmering, tactile sensations that radiates outward in all directions and removes our ability to conceive of ourselves as exclusively solid. While our physical bodies are unable to pass through other physical objects, this dimension of feeling presence, more in the manner of smell that can pass through surfaces, needn't feel so similarly constrained. So convinced are we, though, that matter is exclusively solid that we assume that the surface of an object must be impermeable, and so, if we let our radiance out at all, we tend to let it expand right up to the surface of an object we're looking out at—a book, the wall, another person, anything—but no farther. We believe we can't go any farther and so we stop it there. Instead of allowing the naturally expansive radiance of feeling presence to extend itself ever outward, right through the visual field, maybe even to the far reaches of the universe itself, we dial it way down by bringing tension into our body and mind. We hold ourselves back and our energy in so that we fit more neatly into the container of our beliefs. But conforming to societal expectations through dimming the extent of our radiant expansion ultimately hurts and brings pain to the body, the mind, our deep soul.

From the perspective of form alone, surfaces of objects are indeed opaque. But from the perspective of the great ground of emptiness, this substratum of experience that we all have access to, nothing is opaque. It just looks that way.

What happens when you contact your own innermost essence—empty, spacious, and radiating outward through feeling presence—and then tap into the same dimension of space and emptiness in everything you can perceive at this very moment? What kind of world do you feel out into now?

Shenxiu tells us to constantly tend to the surface of your mind, keeping it clean and free of accumulated dust. Like a gardener, keep removing the weeds as soon as they sprout from the ground so the garden remains pristine.

Hui Neng tells us that since your essential nature is, and always has been, eternally pristine, since the open dimension of being is already existent, there's nothing that you need do to change a thing. Just relax into your nature and one of the things you'll notice is that you dissolve into and through the visual field, altogether naturally, no fuss, no yogic heroics. It's like swimming invisibly through the garden of your vision.

So take your pick—Shenxiu or Hui Neng—but be honest about which approach works for you: Shenxiu, who approaches essential nature through the forms of the world, or Hui Neng, who approaches it directly through the fundamental emptiness of all things. If Hui Neng had a legitimate concern about Shenxiu's obsession with form, Shenxiu could have responded (but didn't—he must have felt completely gobsmacked and was evidently unable to summon a response) with an equally legitimate concern about Hui Neng's obsession with emptiness, and only later would the writer of the Heart Sutra clarify that it isn't a matter of one over the other, but of both somehow existing and being experienced, form as well as emptiness, simultaneously.

Still, the robe and bowl could only go to one person, so the simple lad from the provinces walked away, victorious, with the prize. But what if we focus not on who won or lost but on how the two approaches work together, hand in glove—that if you follow Shenxiu's instructions, you'll reach Hui Neng's gate? And not only do they work together, they complete each other. Form without its underlying dimension of emptiness reveals only half the picture, but emptiness divorced from the world of form promotes an equally illusory vision.

The journey of the dharma is never a one-time event, but something that you will keep repeating every moment of your life. Some moments the larger picture reveals itself in a flashing moment of awareness and you disappear into Hui Neng's great, revitalizing sea of emptiness. Without your having to resort to putting the pieces so painstakingly back together, you simply relax into presence. In other moments you may wake up, like a vessel adrift at sea, to the recognition of how unawake and lost you've become. At those moments, let Shenxiu be your guide; start by feeling the body again and then start relaxing both body and mind, so that mind can turn off its random chatter and start functioning again as a simple, mindful mirror, a mirror deeply fused with its reflections.

The contest might as well have been adjudged a tie, for the subsequent development in Chinese and Japanese Buddhism diverged along two lines, each of which can trace its influence to either Shenxiu's calm and steady approach or Hui Neng's sudden seizing of the moment. In a contest someone has to win and someone has to lose, but might we be better served by embracing the perspectives of both winner and loser, rather than being forced to pick sides?

What happens if you start bringing the body back to felt life and then let yourself look and see the whole of the visual field all at once, as a unified field of appearance? Immediately, thought weakens and body starts to shimmer. And now what happens when you relax and let go completely, allowing bodily presence to expand and radiate outward, as it so wants to do, radiating out farther, right through the surface of appearances, radiating farther even, nothing to stop it, so natural a gesture? Seeing from both Shenxiu's and Hui Neng's perspectives, like two eyes striving for single vision, lets you see both worlds at once, simultaneously, the world of appearances into which you've been born and the invisible world that permeates this one.

Acknowledgments

Special thanks go to Phil Gronquist, who, many long decades ago, first helped me open my eyes and see.

As always, the good folks at Inner Traditions—in particular Jon Graham, Meghan MacLean, Erica Robinson, and Elizabeth Wilson—have been wonderful guides, helpmates, and contributors on this project.

If there was ever an award presented to a spiritual teacher who created a technique of awakening so simple that it was probably destined to be overlooked, that award might easily go to the English seer Douglas Harding. Douglas's book *On Having No Head* inspired me as a young man to pay far more attention to my relationship with the visual field. The Rumi quotation to "dissolve the body into vision" is cited in that book.

To my wonderful wife, Gretavatti, who raises love to the level of devotion, and to my two handsome sons, Kailas and Jamie—all of us fans of the movie *Avatar*—I say, "I see you."

Resources

If you feel drawn to the practice of blowing dust off the mirror, you may want to read the author's

Breathing through the Whole Body
(Inner Traditions, 2012).

If you feel drawn to the practice of eye gazing, you may want to read the author's

The Spiritual Practices of Rumi
(Inner Traditions, 2007)
Rumi's Four Essential Practices
(Inner Traditions, 2010).

Anyone interested in retreats or workshops related to the subject matter of this book may learn more at the author's website, **www.embodiment.net**.

Index

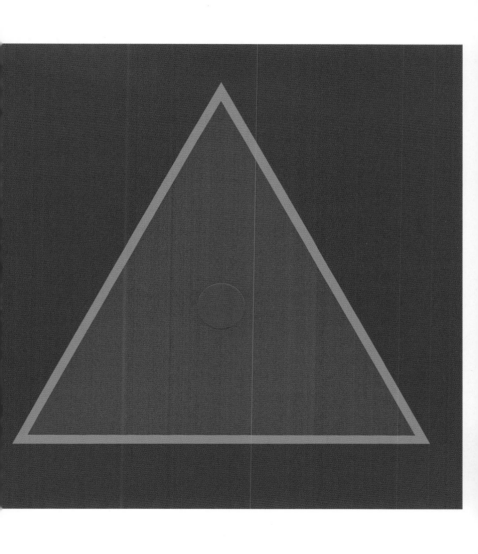

BOOKS OF RELATED INTEREST

Breathing through the Whole Body
The Buddha's Instructions on Integrating Mind, Body, and Breath
by Will Johnson

Yoga of the Mahamudra
The Mystical Way of Balance
by Will Johnson

The Forbidden Rumi
The Suppressed Poems of Rumi on Love, Heresy, and Intoxication
Translations and Commentary by Nevit O. Ergin and Will Johnson

The Rubais of Rumi
Insane with Love
Translations and Commentary by Nevit O. Ergin and Will Johnson

The Spiritual Practices of Rumi
Radical Techniques for Beholding the Divine
by Will Johnson

The Science and Practice of Humility
The Path to Ultimate Freedom
by Jason Gregory
Foreword by Daniel Reid

The Heart of Yoga
Developing a Personal Practice
by T. K. V. Desikachar

The Practice of Tibetan Meditation
Exercises, Visualizations, and Mantras for Health and Well-being
by Dagsay Tulku

INNER TRADITIONS • BEAR & COMPANY
P.O. Box 388
Rochester, VT 05767
1-800-246-8648
www.InnerTraditions.com

Or contact your local bookseller